HIATAL HERNIA

HERNIA

COOKBOOK

SMOOTHIES

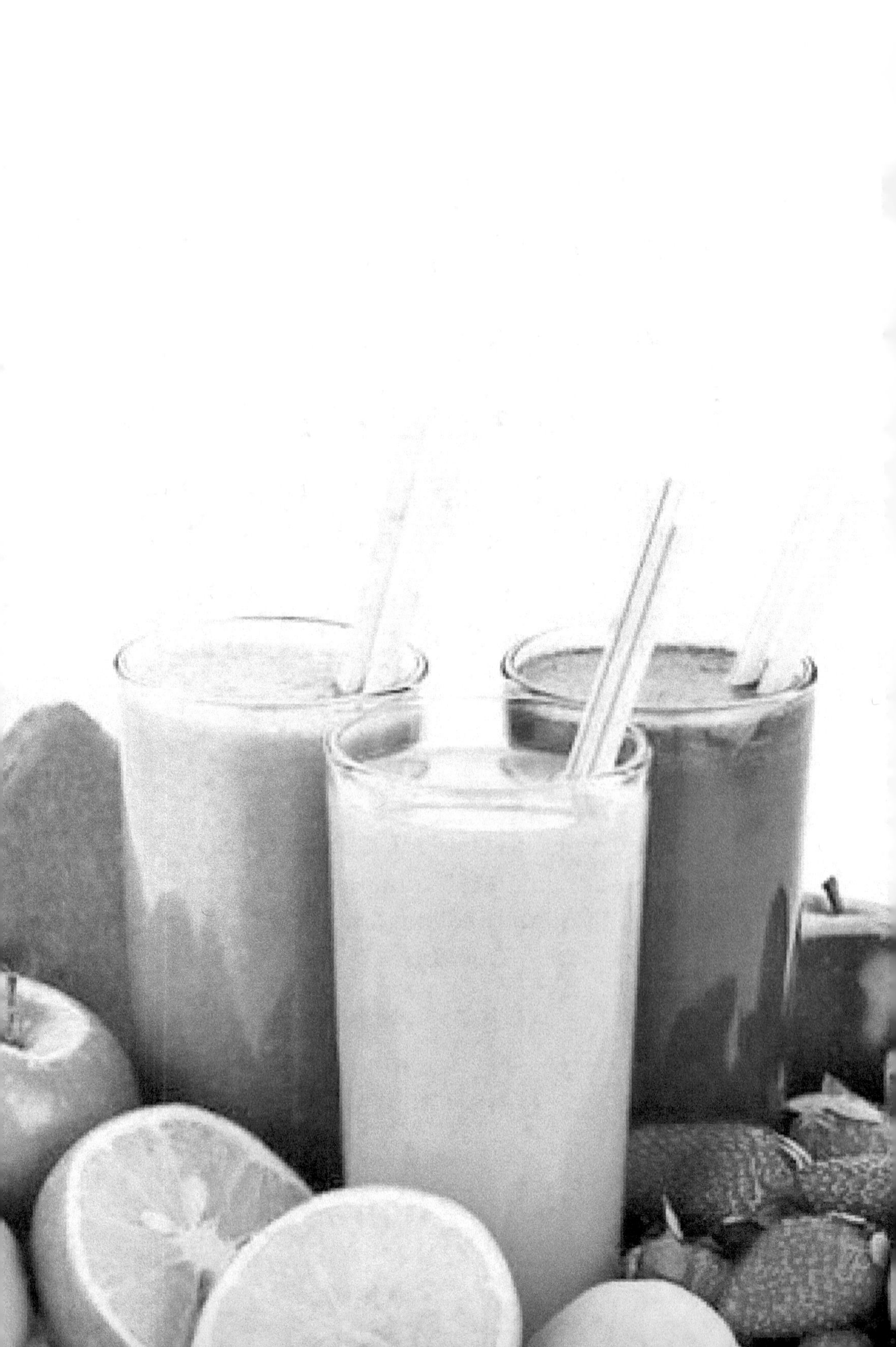

DISCLAIMER:

The information in this book should not be used to diagnose or treat any medical condition. Not every diet and exercise regimen is suitable for everyone. Before beginning any diet, taking any medication, or beginning any fitness or weight-training program, you should always consult with a competent medical expert. The author and publisher expressly disclaim all liability that may arise directly or indirectly from the use of this book. When using kitchen tools, operating ovens and burners, and handling raw food, always use common sense and safety precautions. Readers are encouraged to seek professional assistance when necessary. This guide is provided for informational purposes only, and the author accepts no liability for any liabilities coming from the use of this information.

Printed in the United States of America.

First Edition: February 2024

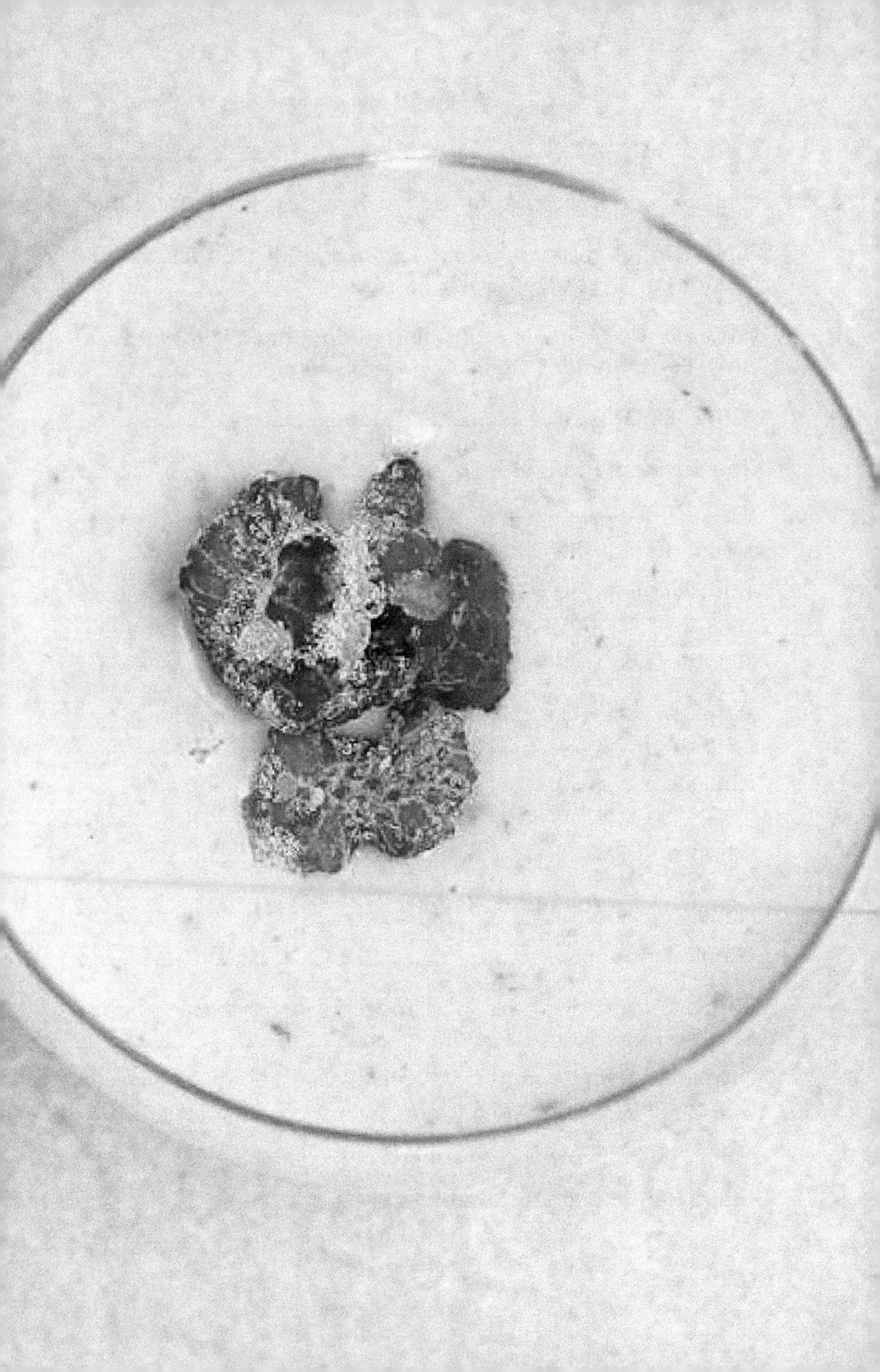

TABLE OF CONTENT

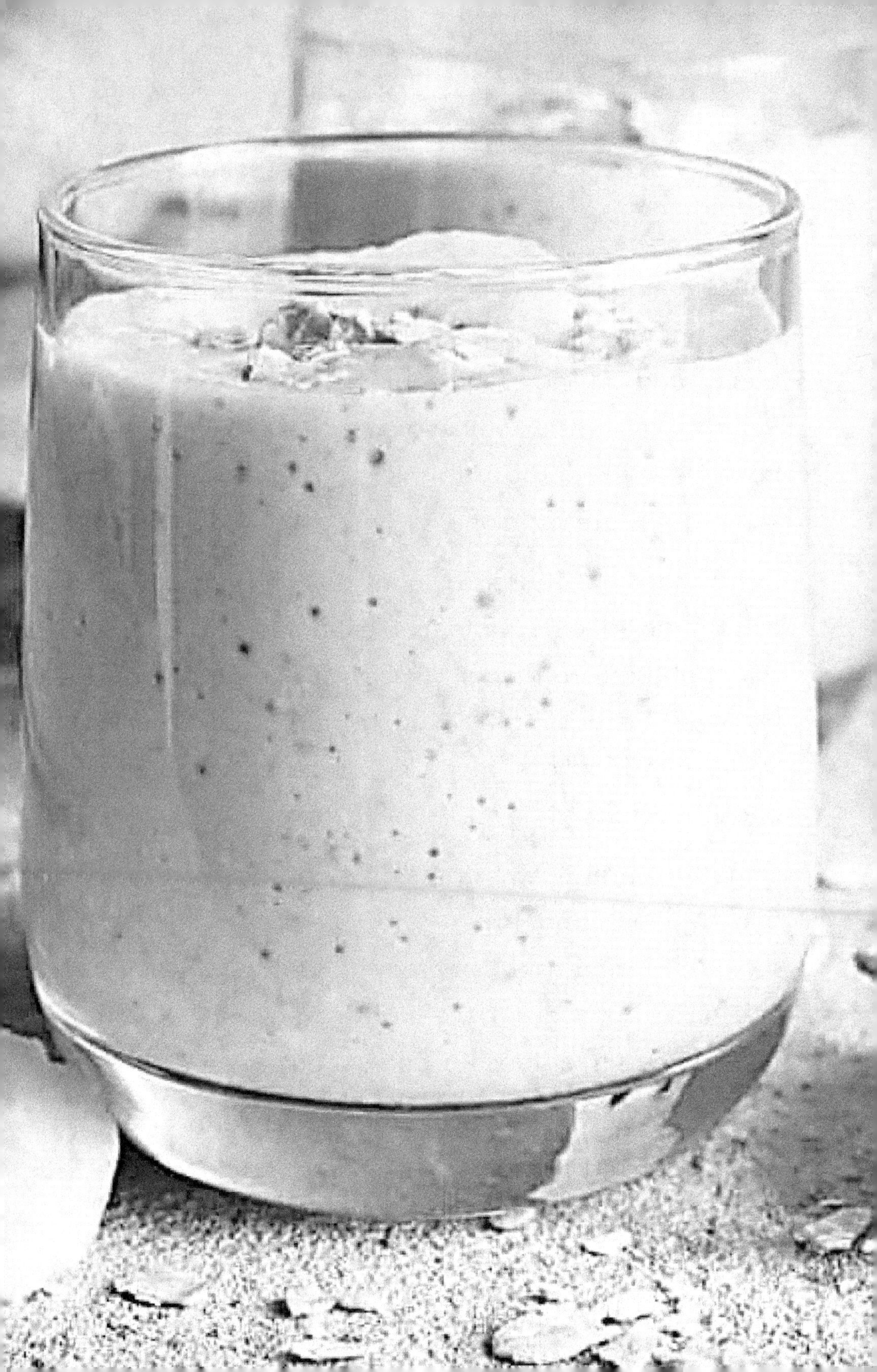

INTRODUCTION

UNLOCKING A HOLISTIC APPROACH TO HEALTH WITH THE DASH DIET

Welcome to the "Hiatal Hernia Cookbook Smoothies," your trusted companion on the journey to reclaiming digestive health and finding relief from the discomfort of Hiatal Hernia symptoms. Whether you're newly diagnosed or have been struggling with this condition for some time, know that you're not alone.

Living with Hiatal Hernia can be challenging, often accompanied by symptoms like heartburn, GERD, and LPR that can significantly impact your quality of life. However, there is hope. Through the power of diet and lifestyle modifications, many individuals have found relief and improved well-being.

In this cookbook, we've gathered a collection of nutritious and delicious smoothie recipes specifically tailored to soothe Hiatal Hernia symptoms and support digestive health. But this book is more than just recipes; it's a source of empathy, understanding, and encouragement.

We understand the frustrations and uncertainties that come with managing Hiatal Hernia. That's why we've included comprehensive guidance on the condition and its symptoms, presented in clear and accessible language. Knowledge is empowering, and we're here to empower you every step of the way.

Throughout these pages, you'll also find personal anecdotes and testimonials from individuals who have successfully managed their Hiatal Hernia symptoms through diet modifications. Their stories serve as a reminder that healing is possible and that you too can find relief.

As you embark on this journey, remember that it's okay to ask for support and seek guidance. You're not alone in this. Together, we'll navigate the challenges of Hiatal Hernia and work towards a future of improved health and well-being.

So, grab your blender and let's embark on this delicious and healing adventure together. Here's to reclaiming your digestive health and living life to the fullest with the "Hiatal Hernia Cookbook Smoothies." Your journey starts now.

Understanding Hiatal Hernia: Explaining the Condition and Its Impact on Digestive Health

Hiatal hernia is a condition that affects millions of people worldwide, yet it remains widely misunderstood. To truly grasp the significance of hiatal hernia, it's essential to first understand its anatomy and mechanics.

At its core, hiatal hernia involves the displacement of the stomach through the diaphragm, specifically through a small opening known as the hiatus. This displacement can occur for various reasons, including genetic predisposition, injury, or prolonged pressure on the abdominal region. As a result, the stomach partially protrudes into the chest cavity, leading to a range of symptoms and complications.

One of the primary impacts of hiatal hernia is its effect on digestive health. The displacement of the stomach can disrupt the natural functioning of the digestive system, leading to issues such as acid reflux, heartburn, and difficulty swallowing. These symptoms not only cause discomfort but can also have a significant impact on daily life, affecting one's ability to eat, sleep, and engage in regular activities.

Moreover, hiatal hernia can exacerbate existing digestive conditions such as gastroesophageal reflux disease

(GERD) and laryngopharyngeal reflux (LPR). The protrusion of the stomach into the chest cavity can weaken the lower esophageal sphincter (LES), allowing stomach acid to reflux into the esophagus and throat, leading to inflammation and irritation.

Beyond the physical symptoms, hiatal hernia can also take a toll on mental and emotional well-being. Living with chronic discomfort and uncertainty about when symptoms will flare up can cause anxiety, stress, and even depression. This aspect of hiatal hernia cannot be overlooked, as mental health plays a significant role in overall quality of life.

Understanding hiatal hernia requires a holistic approach that considers both its physiological mechanisms and its broader impact on well-being. By gaining insight into the condition and its effects on digestive health, individuals can take proactive steps to manage their symptoms and improve their overall quality of life.

Importance of Diet in Managing Hiatal Hernia Symptoms: How Food Choices Can Alleviate Discomfort

When it comes to managing hiatal hernia symptoms, diet plays a crucial role. The foods we consume have a direct impact on digestive health, and making smart dietary choices can help alleviate discomfort and promote healing.

One of the key principles of managing hiatal hernia through diet is to avoid foods that trigger symptoms. These trigger foods can vary from person to person but often include acidic or spicy foods, carbonated beverages, caffeine, chocolate, and fatty or fried foods. By identifying and avoiding these triggers, individuals can minimize the occurrence of symptoms such as heartburn, acid reflux, and indigestion.

In addition to avoiding trigger foods, incorporating hiatal hernia-friendly foods into your diet can help soothe symptoms and promote digestive comfort. These include lean proteins, non-citrus fruits, vegetables, whole grains, and low-fat dairy products. These foods are gentle on the stomach and esophagus, making them ideal choices for individuals with hiatal hernia.

Furthermore, the consistency and texture of foods can also impact hiatal hernia symptoms. Foods that are soft, moist, and easy to swallow are typically better tolerated than hard, dry, or tough foods. Chewing food thoroughly and taking smaller bites can also help prevent discomfort and promote efficient digestion.

Beyond specific food choices, meal timing and portion control are also important considerations for managing hiatal hernia symptoms. Eating smaller, more frequent meals throughout the day can help prevent overloading the stomach and minimize the risk of acid reflux. Additionally, avoiding lying down or going to bed immediately after eating can help prevent nighttime reflux and promote better sleep quality.

Incorporating dietary modifications into your lifestyle may require some trial and error, as what works for one person may not work for another. Keeping a food diary can be helpful in identifying trigger foods and patterns of symptoms, allowing for more targeted dietary adjustments.

Overall, the importance of diet in managing hiatal hernia symptoms cannot be overstated. By making informed food choices, individuals can alleviate discomfort, reduce the frequency and severity of symptoms, and improve their overall quality of life.

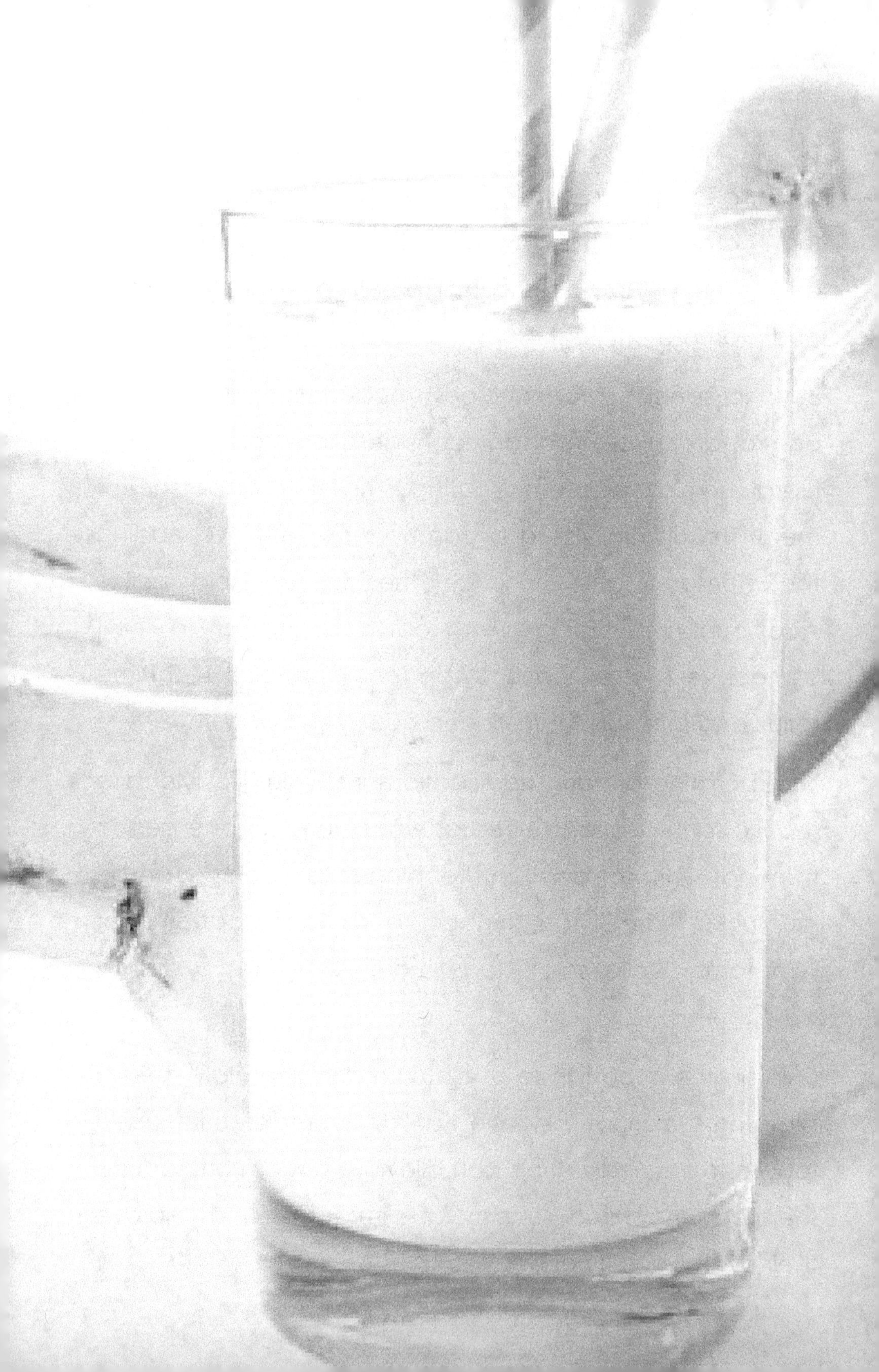

CHAPTER ONE
THE BASICS OF HIATAL HERNIA DIET

What to Eat and What to Avoid: A Comprehensive Guide to Hiatal Hernia-Friendly Foods

Understanding what foods to eat and what to avoid is essential for managing hiatal hernia symptoms and promoting digestive comfort. By making informed dietary choices, individuals can minimize discomfort, reduce the frequency of symptoms, and support overall digestive health.

Hiatal Hernia-Friendly Foods

When it comes to hiatal hernia-friendly foods, the emphasis is on selecting options that are gentle on the stomach, esophagus, and digestive system. Here are some examples of foods that are generally well-tolerated by individuals with hiatal hernia:

1. Lean Proteins: Opt for lean sources of protein such as skinless poultry, fish, tofu, beans, and lentils. These protein sources are easier to digest and less likely to trigger symptoms like acid reflux.

2. **Non-Citrus Fruits:** Choose non-acidic fruits such as bananas, apples, pears, melons, and berries. These fruits provide essential nutrients and fiber without exacerbating acid reflux or heartburn.

3. **Vegetables:** Incorporate a variety of vegetables into your diet, focusing on non-acidic options like leafy greens, broccoli, carrots, zucchini, and squash. Vegetables are rich in vitamins, minerals, and antioxidants, promoting overall digestive health.

4. **Whole Grains:** Opt for whole grains such as oats, brown rice, quinoa, barley, and whole wheat bread or pasta. Whole grains are high in fiber, which aids in digestion and helps prevent constipation.

5. **Low-Fat Dairy Products:** Choose low-fat or non-fat dairy products such as milk, yogurt, and cheese. These dairy options provide calcium and protein without excessive fat content, reducing the risk of triggering symptoms.

6. **Healthy Fats:** Include sources of healthy fats in your diet such as avocados, nuts, seeds, and olive oil. These fats provide essential nutrients and support overall health without aggravating digestive discomfort.

Foods to Avoid

While certain foods are beneficial for individuals with hiatal hernia, others can exacerbate symptoms and should be avoided or limited. Here are some examples of foods to avoid:

1. **Acidic Foods:** Steer clear of acidic foods and beverages such as citrus fruits, tomatoes, citrus juices, vinegar, and carbonated drinks. These acidic foods can irritate the esophagus and trigger symptoms like heartburn and acid reflux.

2. **Spicy Foods:** Limit or avoid spicy foods and dishes containing hot peppers, chili powder, garlic, and onions. Spicy foods can increase stomach acid production and exacerbate symptoms of acid reflux and indigestion.

3. **Fatty or Fried Foods:** Avoid high-fat and fried foods such as fried chicken, French fries, fatty cuts of

meat, and creamy sauces. These foods can relax the lower esophageal sphincter (LES) and delay stomach emptying, leading to increased acid reflux and discomfort.

4. **Chocolate and Caffeine:** Limit or avoid chocolate and caffeinated beverages such as coffee, tea, and soda. Both chocolate and caffeine can relax the LES and stimulate stomach acid production, contributing to symptoms of acid reflux and heartburn.

5. **Mint and Peppermint:** Steer clear of mint and peppermint products, including peppermint tea and mint-flavored candies. Mint can relax the LES and worsen symptoms of acid reflux and indigestion.

6. **Alcohol and Tobacco:** Reduce or eliminate alcohol and tobacco consumption, as both can weaken the LES and increase the risk of acid reflux and digestive discomfort.

By being mindful of your food choices and avoiding trigger foods, you can minimize symptoms of hiatal hernia and support your digestive health. Experiment with different foods to see how your body responds and adjust your diet accordingly. Remember to focus on whole, nutrient-dense foods and prioritize balance and moderation in your eating habits.

Tips for Eating Well with Hiatal Hernia: Portion Control, Meal Timing, and Eating Habits

In addition to selecting hiatal hernia-friendly foods, adopting healthy eating habits and practices can further support digestive comfort and symptom management. Here are some tips for eating well with hiatal hernia:

Portion Control

Practicing portion control is crucial for individuals with hiatal hernia, as overeating can increase pressure on the stomach and exacerbate symptoms like acid reflux and heartburn. Here are some strategies for controlling portion sizes:

1. Use smaller plates and bowls to help control portion sizes and prevent overeating.

2. Pay attention to hunger and fullness cues, stopping eating when you feel satisfied rather than overly full.

3. Divide your plate into sections, with vegetables taking up the largest portion, followed by lean protein and whole grains.

4. Avoid going back for seconds or eating directly from large packages or containers, as this can lead to mindless eating and overconsumption.

Meal Timing

The timing of meals and snacks can also impact hiatal hernia symptoms. By spacing out meals and snacks throughout the day and avoiding eating close to bedtime, you can reduce the risk of experiencing nighttime reflux and discomfort. Here are some tips for optimizing meal timing:

1. Aim to eat smaller, more frequent meals throughout the day rather than a few large meals. This can help prevent overloading the stomach and minimize the risk of acid reflux.

2. Allow at least two to three hours between your last meal or snack and bedtime to allow for adequate digestion and reduce the likelihood of nighttime reflux.

3. If you experience symptoms of acid reflux or heartburn at night, consider elevating the head of your bed or sleeping with an extra pillow to keep your upper body elevated.

Eating Habits

In addition to portion control and meal timing, adopting healthy eating habits can promote digestive comfort and minimize symptoms of hiatal hernia. Here are some eating habits to consider:

1. Chew food thoroughly and eat slowly to aid digestion and prevent swallowing air, which can contribute to bloating and gas.

2. Sit upright while eating and avoid lying down or reclining immediately after meals, as this can increase pressure on the stomach and lead to reflux.

3. Take time to enjoy your meals and savor the flavors, textures, and aromas of your food. Mindful eating can help you feel more satisfied and prevent overeating.

4. Stay hydrated by drinking plenty of water throughout the day, but avoid drinking large

amounts of liquid with meals, as this can dilute stomach acid and impair digestion.

By practicing portion control, optimizing meal timing, and adopting healthy eating habits, you can support digestive comfort and minimize symptoms of hiatal hernia. Remember to listen to your body and adjust as needed to find what works best for you. With mindful eating practices and a focus on hiatal hernia-friendly foods, you can take control of your digestive health and improve your overall well-being.

.

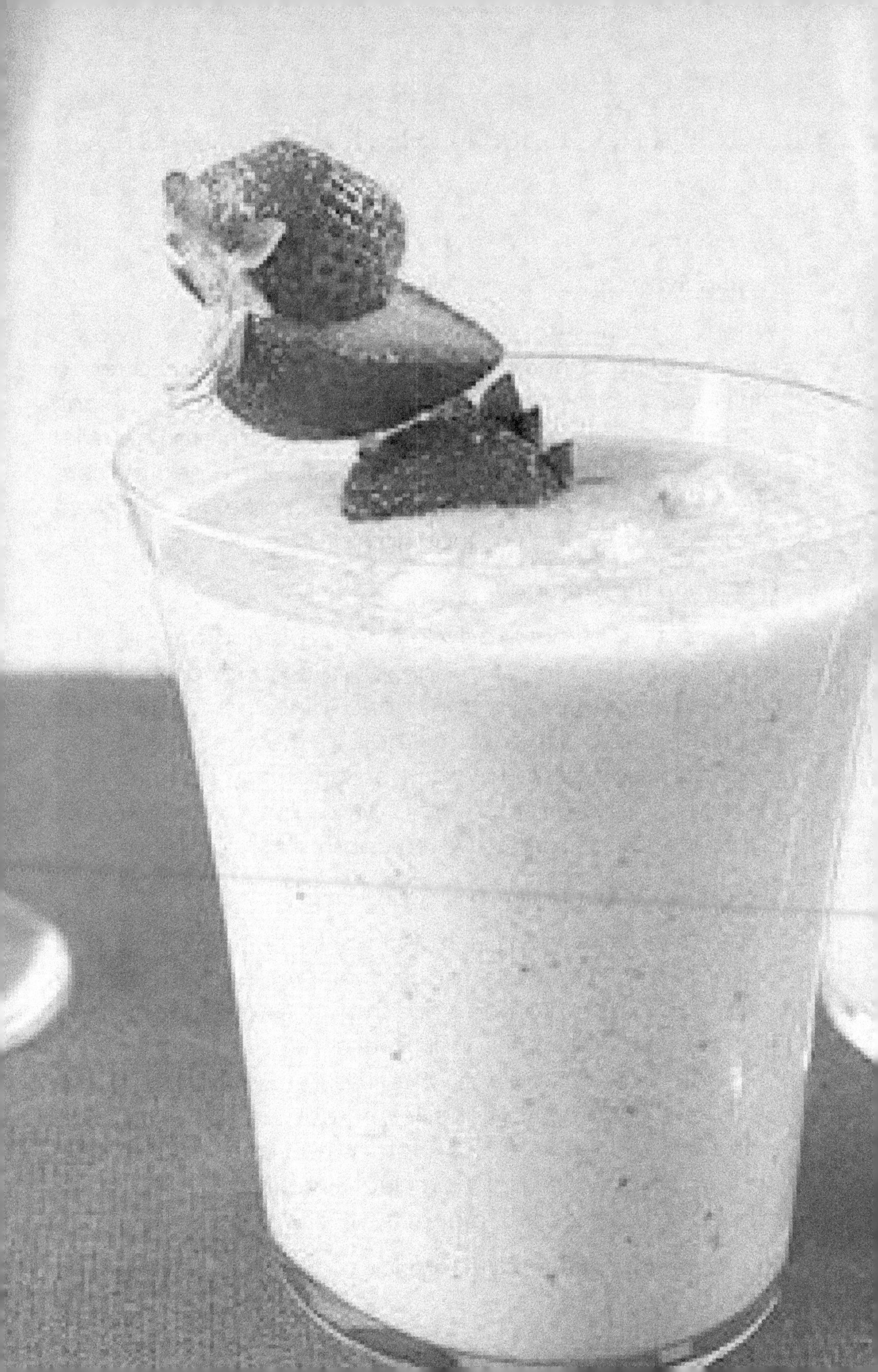

CHAPTER TWO
BENEFITS OF SMOOTHIES FOR HIATAL HERNIA

Why Smoothies are a Great Option for Managing Hiatal Hernia Symptoms

When it comes to managing hiatal hernia symptoms, incorporating smoothies into your diet can offer a multitude of benefits. Smoothies are a convenient, versatile, and easy-to-digest option that can provide relief from discomfort and support overall digestive health. Here are several reasons why smoothies are an excellent choice for individuals managing hiatal hernia:

Gentle on the Stomach

One of the primary advantages of smoothies is their gentle nature on the stomach. Unlike solid foods that may require more effort to chew and digest, smoothies are blended into a liquid form, making them easier for the stomach to process. This can be particularly beneficial for individuals with hiatal hernia who may have trouble swallowing or discomfort when consuming solid foods.

Customizable Ingredients

Another advantage of smoothies is their flexibility and versatility. With a wide range of ingredients to choose from, you can customize your smoothie to suit your taste preferences and nutritional needs. Whether you prefer fruity, creamy, or savory flavors, there's a smoothie recipe out there for you. Additionally, you can easily incorporate hiatal hernia-friendly foods such as non-acidic fruits, leafy greens, and low-fat dairy products into your smoothies to maximize their digestive benefits.

Hydration and Nutrient Absorption

Smoothies are an excellent way to stay hydrated while also boosting your nutrient intake. By blending fruits and vegetables with water, juice, or milk, you can create a hydrating beverage that replenishes fluids and electrolytes lost throughout the day. Furthermore, the blended nature of smoothies can enhance nutrient absorption, allowing your body to more efficiently extract vitamins, minerals, and antioxidants from the ingredients.

Portability and Convenience

Smoothies are an ideal option for individuals with busy lifestyles or on-the-go schedules. Whether you're rushing out the door in the morning or need a quick and nutritious snack between meals, smoothies can be prepared ahead of time and enjoyed anytime, anywhere. Simply blend your ingredients, pour into a portable container, and you're ready to take your smoothie with you wherever you go.

Promotes Satiety and Weight Management

Smoothies can be a satisfying and filling option that can help curb cravings and promote weight management. By incorporating ingredients high in fiber, protein, and healthy fats, such as fruits, vegetables, nuts, seeds, and Greek yogurt, you can create a nutrient-dense smoothie that keeps you feeling full and satisfied for longer. Additionally, the liquid nature of smoothies can help promote hydration, which is essential for maintaining a healthy weight.

Reduced Risk of Acid Reflux

For individuals with hiatal hernia, acid reflux and heartburn are common symptoms that can be exacerbated by certain foods and beverages. Smoothies offer a convenient and customizable option that allows you to enjoy a variety of flavors and nutrients without the risk of triggering acid reflux. By selecting hiatal hernia-friendly ingredients and avoiding acidic or spicy additives, you can minimize the likelihood of experiencing discomfort while still nourishing your body.

Overall, smoothies are a fantastic option for individuals managing hiatal hernia symptoms. They offer a convenient, customizable, and gentle way to stay hydrated, boost nutrient intake, promote satiety, and minimize the risk of acid reflux. By incorporating smoothies into your diet regularly, you can support your digestive health and enhance your overall well-being.

Nutritional Benefits of Smoothies: Boosting Nutrient Intake and Supporting Digestive Health

Smoothies are not only delicious and refreshing but also pack a powerful nutritional punch. By blending, a variety of fruits, vegetables, protein sources, and other nutrient-rich ingredients, smoothies offer a convenient and efficient way to boost your nutrient intake and support digestive health. Here are several nutritional benefits of incorporating smoothies into your diet:

Rich in Vitamins and Minerals

Fruits and vegetables are naturally rich in essential vitamins and minerals that are vital for overall health and well-being. By blending a variety of colorful fruits and vegetables into your smoothies, you can ensure you're getting a wide range of nutrients, including vitamin C, vitamin A, potassium, magnesium, and folate. These nutrients play key roles in supporting immune function, promoting healthy skin and hair, maintaining bone health, and supporting overall vitality.

High in Fiber

Fiber is an important nutrient that plays a crucial role in digestive health. It helps regulate bowel movements, prevent constipation, and support the growth of beneficial gut bacteria. By including fiber-rich ingredients such as fruits, vegetables, nuts, seeds, and whole grains in your smoothies, you can increase your fiber intake and promote optimal digestion. Additionally, fiber helps promote feelings of fullness and satiety, which can aid in weight management and prevent overeating.

Provides Antioxidants

Antioxidants are compounds found in certain foods that help protect the body from oxidative stress and inflammation. They neutralize harmful free radicals, which can damage cells and contribute to chronic diseases such as heart disease, cancer, and diabetes. Many fruits and vegetables are rich in antioxidants such as vitamins C and E, beta-carotene, and flavonoids. By including antioxidant-rich ingredients like berries, leafy greens, and citrus fruits in your smoothies, you can help reduce inflammation, support immune function, and promote overall health and longevity.

Supports Hydration

Proper hydration is essential for overall health and well-being. Smoothies provide a convenient and delicious way to stay hydrated, especially when blended with water, juice, or milk. Fruits and vegetables have high water content, which helps replenish fluids and electrolytes lost through sweat, urine, and respiration. By sipping on smoothies throughout the day, you can maintain optimal hydration levels and support various bodily functions, including digestion, circulation, temperature regulation, and nutrient transport.

Aids in Digestion and Gut Health

Smoothies can help support digestive health by providing a concentrated source of nutrients that are easy to digest and absorb. Blending fruits and vegetables breaks down their cell walls, making it easier for the body to access and utilize the nutrients they contain. Additionally, smoothies can help promote the growth of beneficial gut bacteria, which play a crucial role in digestion, nutrient absorption, and immune function. By including probiotic-rich ingredients such as yogurt, kefir, and fermented foods in your smoothies, you can support a healthy balance of gut bacteria and improve overall digestive health.

Promotes Weight Management

Smoothies can be a valuable tool for individuals looking to manage their weight or support weight loss goals. By incorporating nutrient-dense ingredients such as fruits, vegetables, protein sources, and healthy fats into your smoothies, you can create a filling and satisfying meal or snack that helps curb cravings and prevent overeating. Additionally, the liquid nature of smoothies can help promote feelings of fullness and satiety, making them an excellent option for those looking to control portion sizes and reduce overall calorie intake.

In summary, smoothies offer a wide range of nutritional benefits that can help support overall health and well-being. By incorporating a variety of fruits, vegetables, protein sources, and other nutrient-rich ingredients into your smoothies, you can boost your nutrient intake, support digestive health, promote hydration, and aid in weight management. Whether enjoyed as a meal replacement, post-workout refresher, or nutritious snack, smoothies are a delicious and convenient way to nourish your body and enhance your vitality.

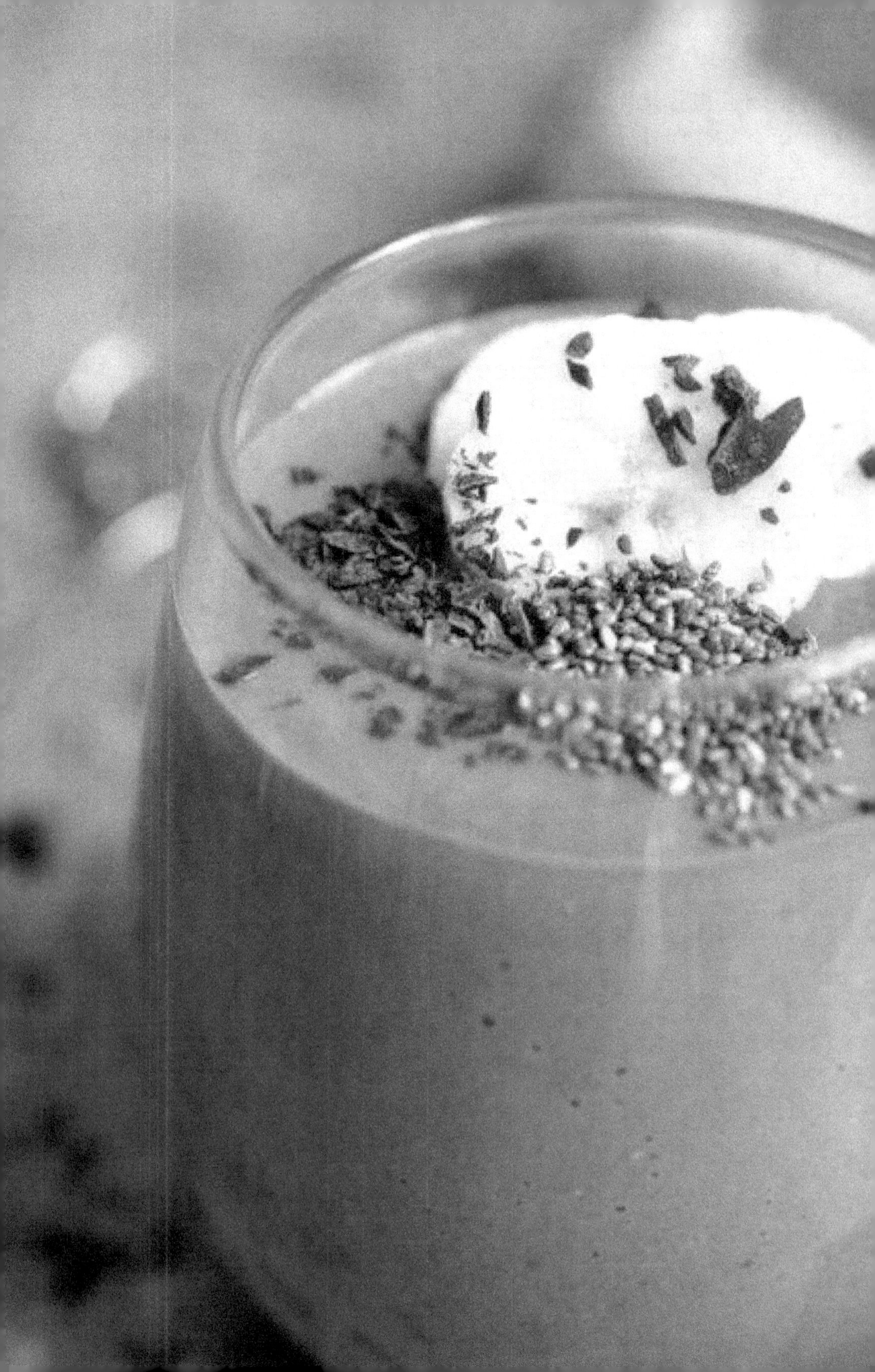

CHAPTER THREE
ESSENTIAL INGREDIENTS FOR HIATAL HERNIA SMOOTHIES

Building Blocks of a Nutritious Smoothie: Incorporating Healing Ingredients and Superfoods

When it comes to crafting smoothies for hiatal hernia, choosing the right ingredients is key to maximizing their digestive benefits and promoting overall well-being. By incorporating healing ingredients and superfoods into your smoothies, you can create delicious and nourishing beverages that support digestive health and alleviate discomfort. Here are some essential ingredients to consider including in your hiatal hernia smoothies:

Leafy Greens

Leafy greens such as spinach, kale, Swiss chard, and collard greens are nutritional powerhouses packed with vitamins, minerals, and antioxidants. These greens are rich in fiber, which helps promote digestion and regulate bowel movements. Additionally, leafy greens contain compounds like chlorophyll and phytonutrients that have anti-inflammatory and detoxifying properties, making them excellent choices for individuals with hiatal hernia.

Non-Acidic Fruits

When selecting fruits for your hiatal hernia smoothies, opt for non-acidic options that are less likely to trigger acid reflux or heartburn. Some examples of non-acidic fruits include bananas, apples, pears, mangoes, and berries. These fruits provide essential vitamins, minerals, and antioxidants without exacerbating digestive discomfort.

Additionally, their natural sweetness adds delicious flavor and texture to your smoothies.

Low-Fat Dairy or Dairy Alternatives

Dairy products such as yogurt and kefir are rich sources of probiotics, beneficial bacteria that support digestive health and promote a healthy gut microbiome. However, individuals with lactose intolerance or dairy sensitivities may need to opt for dairy-free alternatives such as almond milk, coconut milk, or soy milk. These dairy alternatives are typically lower in fat and lactose, making them easier to digest and suitable for individuals with hiatal hernia.

Healthy Fats

Incorporating healthy fats into your smoothies can help promote satiety, stabilize blood sugar levels, and support overall digestive health. Some examples of healthy fats to include in your hiatal hernia smoothies include avocados, nuts, seeds, and nut butters. These fats provide essential fatty acids such as omega-3s and omega-6s, which have anti-inflammatory properties and support heart health.

Protein Sources

Adding protein to your smoothies can help promote satiety, support muscle repair and growth, and stabilize blood sugar levels. Some protein-rich ingredients to include in your hiatal hernia smoothies include Greek yogurt, tofu, protein powder (such as whey, pea, or hemp protein), and nut or seed butters. Be mindful of choosing lean protein sources and avoiding highly processed protein powders with added sugars and artificial ingredients.

Herbs and Spices

Herbs and spices not only add flavor and depth to your smoothies but also provide a wide range of health benefits. Some herbs and spices that are particularly beneficial for digestive health include ginger, turmeric, cinnamon, and mint. These herbs and spices have anti-inflammatory, anti-nausea, and digestive-stimulating properties, making them excellent additions to hiatal hernia smoothies.

Fiber-Rich Ingredients

Fiber is essential for promoting digestive health and regulating bowel movements. Including fiber-rich ingredients such as flaxseeds, chia seeds, oats, and psyllium husk in your hiatal hernia smoothies can help promote feelings of fullness, support regularity, and prevent constipation. Additionally, fiber helps slow down the digestion and absorption of carbohydrates, which can help stabilize blood sugar levels and prevent spikes in insulin.

Hydration Enhancers

Staying hydrated is crucial for supporting overall health and well-being, especially for individuals with hiatal hernia. Adding hydrating ingredients such as coconut water, cucumber, celery, and watermelon to your smoothies can help replenish fluids and electrolytes lost through sweating, urination, and respiration. These ingredients also provide essential vitamins, minerals, and antioxidants that support hydration and overall health.

Incorporating these essential ingredients into your hiatal hernia smoothies can help maximize their digestive benefits and promote overall well-being. Experiment with different combinations and ratios to find the flavors and textures that appeal to you most. Whether enjoyed as a meal replacement, post-workout refresher, or nutritious snack, hiatal hernia smoothies offer a convenient and delicious way to support digestive health and alleviate discomfort.

Substitutions for Common Smoothie Ingredients: Catering to Dietary Restrictions and Preferences

When creating smoothies for hiatal hernia, it's important to consider individual dietary restrictions and preferences. Fortunately, many common smoothie ingredients can be easily substituted to accommodate various dietary needs while still maintaining flavor, texture, and nutritional value. Here are some substitutions for common smoothie ingredients to help you cater to dietary restrictions and preferences:

Dairy Substitutions

For individuals with lactose intolerance or dairy sensitivities, dairy-free alternatives can be used in place of traditional dairy products. Almond milk, coconut milk, soy milk, and oat milk are popular dairy-free options that provide similar creaminess and texture to cow's milk. Additionally, dairy-free yogurt and kefir made from coconut, almond, or soy can be used as substitutes for traditional yogurt and kefir in smoothie recipes.

Protein Powder Alternatives

While whey protein powder is a popular choice for adding protein to smoothies, there are plenty of plant based protein powders available for individuals following a vegetarian, vegan, or dairy-free diet. Pea protein, hemp protein, rice protein, and soy protein are all viable alternatives to whey protein powder and can be used in smoothie recipes to boost protein content without compromising flavor or texture.

Sweeteners

Many smoothie recipes call for added sweeteners such as honey, maple syrup, or agave nectar to enhance flavor. However, individuals looking to reduce their sugar intake or avoid refined sugars can opt for natural sweeteners such as dates, bananas, or stevia instead. These natural sweeteners provide sweetness without causing spikes in blood sugar levels and can be used in moderation to sweeten smoothies to taste.

Gluten-Free Options

For individuals with celiac disease or gluten sensitivity, it's important to choose gluten-free ingredients when preparing smoothies. Gluten-free grains such as quinoa, oats, and buckwheat can be used as substitutes for wheat-based ingredients like wheat germ or wheat bran. Additionally, gluten-free protein powders made from pea, rice, or hemp protein are available for individuals seeking gluten-free options for their smoothies.

Low-FODMAP Choices

For individuals with irritable bowel syndrome (IBS) or other gastrointestinal disorders, following a low-FODMAP diet can help alleviate digestive symptoms. FODMAPs are fermentable carbohydrates found in certain foods that can trigger digestive issues in sensitive individuals. When creating smoothies for individuals following a low-FODMAP diet, it's important to choose ingredients that are low in FODMAPs. Some low-FODMAP options include bananas, strawberries, blueberries, spinach, lactose-free yogurt, and almond milk.

Allergen-Free Ingredients

Individuals with food allergies must be vigilant about avoiding allergens in their diet, including in smoothie recipes. Common food allergens include peanuts, tree nuts, eggs, soy, wheat, dairy, fish, and shellfish. When preparing smoothies for individuals with food allergies, it's essential to carefully read ingredient labels and choose allergen-free alternatives. For example, sunflower seed butter can be used as a substitute for peanut butter, and coconut yogurt can be used as a substitute for dairy yogurt in allergen-free smoothie recipes.

By making thoughtful substitutions and adjustments, you can create delicious and nutritious smoothies that cater to a wide range of dietary restrictions and preferences. Whether you're following a dairy-free, gluten-free, low-FODMAP, or allergen-free diet, there are plenty of options available to help you enjoy smoothies while supporting your digestive health and overall well-being. Experiment with different ingredients and combinations to find the perfect smoothie recipe that meets your dietary needs and tastes delicious.

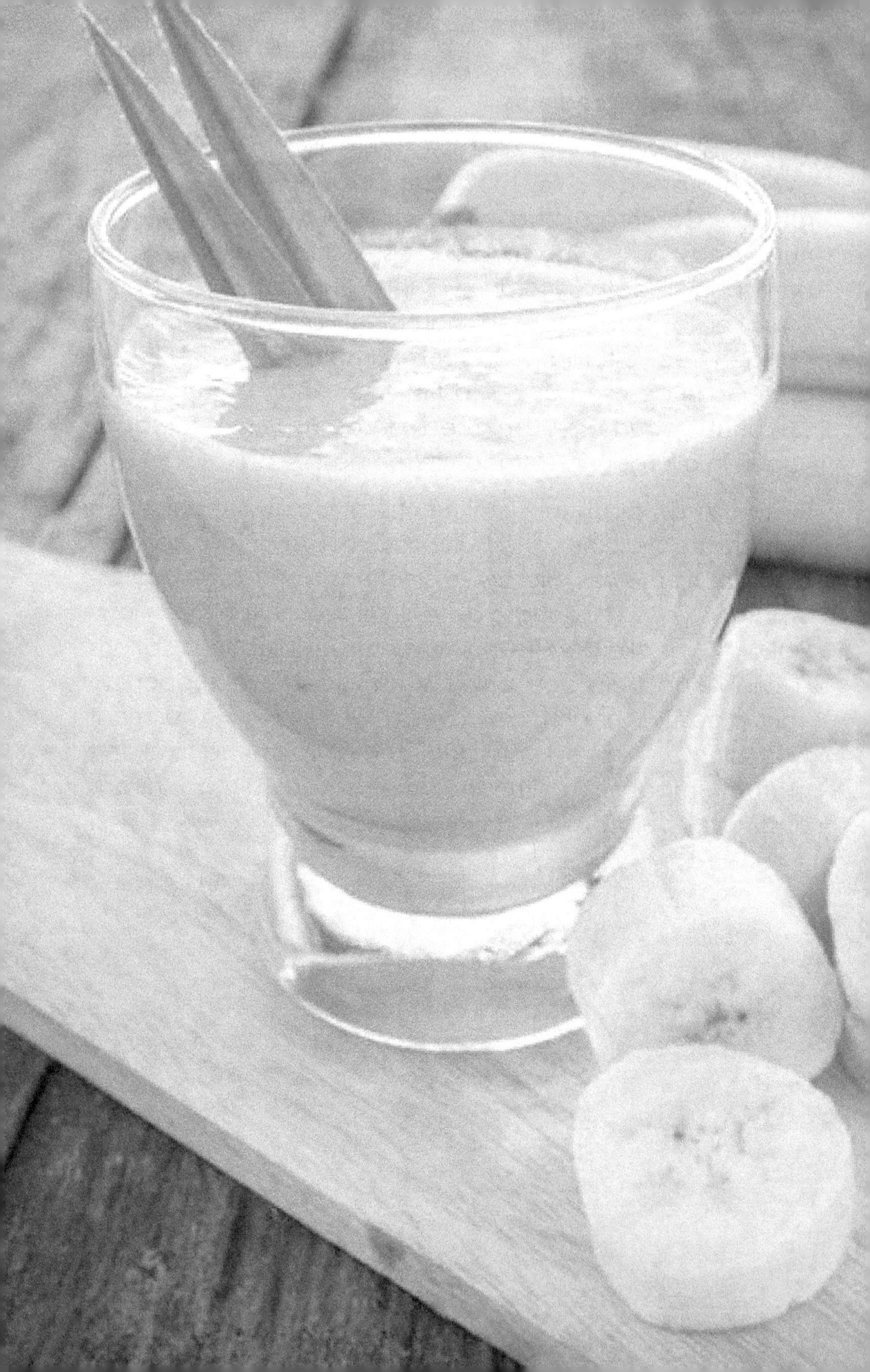

CHAPTER FOUR

HIATAL HERNIA-FRIENDLY SMOOTHIE RECIPES

Gentle Green Smoothie: Soothing Blend for Sensitive Stomachs

As a registered dietitian specializing in digestive health, I understand the importance of gentle and soothing foods for individuals managing hiatal hernia symptoms. These gentle green smoothie variations are designed to be easy on the stomach while providing essential nutrients to support digestive health and alleviate discomfort. Each recipe incorporates hiatal hernia-friendly ingredients that are gentle, nourishing, and delicious.

1. Simple Spinach Smoothie

Ingredients:

- 1 cup fresh spinach leaves
- 1 ripe banana
- 1/2 cup cucumber, chopped
- 1/2 cup coconut water
- 1 tablespoon fresh ginger, grated
- Optional: 1 tablespoon honey or maple syrup for sweetness

Instructions:

1. Combine all ingredients in a blender.
2. Blend until smooth and creamy.
3. Taste and adjust sweetness if desired by adding honey or maple syrup.

4. Pour into a glass and enjoy immediately.

2. Creamy Avocado Kale Smoothie

Ingredients:

- 1 cup kale leaves, stems removed
- 1/2 ripe avocado
- 1/2 cup pineapple chunks
- 1/2 cup almond milk (or dairy-free milk of choice)
- 1 tablespoon chia seeds
- Optional: 1 tablespoon honey or maple syrup for sweetness

Instructions:

1. Place all ingredients in a blender.
2. Blend until creamy and smooth.
3. Taste and add honey or maple syrup if desired for sweetness.
4. Pour into a glass and serve chilled.

3. Cooling Cucumber Mint Smoothie

Ingredients:

- 1 cup cucumber, peeled and chopped
- 1/2 cup fresh spinach leaves
- 1/4 cup fresh mint leaves
- 1/2 cup Greek yogurt (or dairy-free yogurt)
- 1/2 cup coconut water
- Optional: 1 tablespoon honey or maple syrup for sweetness

Instructions:

1. Combine all ingredients in a blender.

2. Blend until well combined and smooth.

3. Taste and adjust sweetness with honey or maple syrup if desired.

4. Pour into glasses and garnish with fresh mint leaves.

4. Banana Berry Blast Smoothie

Ingredients:

- 1 ripe banana
- 1/2 cup mixed berries (such as strawberries, blueberries, raspberries)
- 1/2 cup spinach leaves
- 1/2 cup almond milk (or dairy-free milk of choice)
- 1 tablespoon flaxseed meal
- Optional: 1 tablespoon honey or maple syrup for sweetness

Instructions:

1. Place all ingredients in a blender.

2. Blend until smooth and creamy.

3. Taste and add honey or maple syrup if desired for sweetness.

4. Pour into glasses and serve immediately.

5. Tropical Turmeric Smoothie

Ingredients:

- 1/2 cup frozen mango chunks
- 1/2 cup fresh spinach leaves
- 1/2 teaspoon ground turmeric

- 1/2 teaspoon ground cinnamon

- 1/2 cup coconut water

- 1/2 cup Greek yogurt (or dairy-free yogurt)

- Optional: 1 tablespoon honey or maple syrup for sweetness

Instructions:

1. Add all ingredients to a blender.

2. Blend until smooth and creamy.

3. Taste and adjust sweetness with honey or maple syrup if desired.

4. Pour into glasses and serve chilled.

These gentle green smoothie variations are perfect for individuals with hiatal hernia or sensitive stomachs. Packed with nutrient-rich ingredients and soothing flavors, these smoothies provide a refreshing and nourishing option for supporting digestive health and promoting overall well-being. Enjoy these smoothies as a nutritious breakfast, snack, or post-workout refresher, and feel confident knowing you're giving your body the care and nourishment it deserves.

Berry Banana Bliss: Antioxidant-Rich and Digestive-Friendly Delight

As a registered dietitian specializing in digestive health, I've crafted these Berry Banana Bliss smoothie variations to provide both delicious flavor and digestive support for individuals managing hiatal hernia symptoms. These smoothies are packed with antioxidant-rich berries and soothing banana, making them gentle on the stomach while promoting overall well-being. Enjoy these delightful smoothies any time of day for a nourishing boost of nutrients.

1. Classic Berry Banana Blend

Ingredients:

- 1 ripe banana
- 1/2 cup mixed berries (such as strawberries, blueberries, raspberries)
- 1/2 cup spinach leaves
- 1/2 cup almond milk (or dairy-free milk of choice)
- 1 tablespoon flaxseed meal

Instructions:

1. Place all ingredients in a blender.
2. Blend until smooth and creamy.
3. Pour into glasses and enjoy immediately.

Nutritional Information (per serving):

- Calories: 150
- Protein: 4g
- Fat: 4g

- Carbohydrates: 28g

- Fiber: 6g

- Sugars: 15g

Ingredients:

- 1 ripe banana

- 1/2 cup mixed berries (such as strawberries, blueberries, raspberries)

- 1/2 cup pineapple chunks

- 1/2 cup spinach leaves

- 1/2 cup coconut water

Instructions:

1. Add all ingredients to a blender.

2. Blend until smooth and creamy.

3. Pour into glasses and garnish with a pineapple slice if desired.

Nutritional Information (per serving):

- Calories: 170

- Protein: 3g

- Fat: 1g

- Carbohydrates: 40g

- Fiber: 7g

- Sugars: 24g

3. Berry Banana Protein Powerhouse

Ingredients:

- 1 ripe banana
- 1/2 cup mixed berries (such as strawberries, blueberries, raspberries)
- 1/2 cup spinach leaves
- 1/2 cup Greek yogurt (or dairy-free yogurt)
- 1 tablespoon almond butter
- 1 tablespoon chia seeds

Instructions:

1. Combine all ingredients in a blender.
2. Blend until smooth and creamy.
3. Pour into glasses and top with additional chia seeds for added texture and nutrients.

Nutritional Information (per serving):

- Calories: 250
- Protein: 12g
- Fat: 10g
- Carbohydrates: 30g
- Fiber: 8g
- Sugars: 15g

4. Berry Banana Green Goddess

Ingredients:

- 1 ripe banana
- 1/2 cup mixed berries (such as strawberries, blueberries, raspberries)
- 1/2 cup spinach leaves
- 1/2 cup cucumber, chopped
- 1/2 cup coconut water
- 1 tablespoon fresh mint leaves

Instructions:

1. Place all ingredients in a blender.
2. Blend until smooth and creamy.
3. Pour into glasses and garnish with a mint sprig for a refreshing touch.

Nutritional Information (per serving):

- Calories: 120
- Protein: 3g
- Fat: 1g
- Carbohydrates: 25g
- Fiber: 5g
- Sugars: 14g

5. Berry Banana Immunity Booster

Ingredients:

- 1 ripe banana
- 1/2 cup mixed berries (such as strawberries, blueberries, raspberries)
- 1/2 cup spinach leaves
- 1/2 cup orange juice (freshly squeezed if possible)
- 1/2 teaspoon grated ginger
- 1/4 teaspoon ground turmeric

Instructions:

1. Add all ingredients to a blender.
2. Blend until smooth and creamy.
3. Pour into glasses and enjoy this immune-boosting smoothie to support overall health and vitality.

Nutritional Information (per serving):

- Calories: 160
- Protein: 3g
- Fat: 1g
- Carbohydrates: 35g
- Fiber: 6g
- Sugars: 20g

These Berry Banana Bliss smoothie variations provide a delicious and nutritious way to support digestive health and promote overall well-being. Enjoy the antioxidant-rich blend of berries and banana in each sip, knowing you're nourishing your body with essential nutrients and gentle ingredients.

Creamy Coconut Pineapple: Tropical Treat for Hiatal Hernia Management

As a registered dietitian specializing in digestive health, I've developed these Creamy Coconut Pineapple smoothie variations to offer a delicious and soothing option for individuals managing hiatal hernia symptoms. Packed with tropical flavors and gentle ingredients, these smoothies are designed to support digestive comfort and overall well-being. Enjoy these refreshing tropical treats any time of day for a nourishing boost of nutrients.

1. Classic Coconut Pineapple Bliss

Ingredients:

- 1/2 cup pineapple chunks (fresh or frozen)
- 1/2 ripe banana
- 1/2 cup spinach leaves
- 1/2 cup coconut milk
- 1/4 cup Greek yogurt (or dairy-free yogurt)
- 1 tablespoon honey or maple syrup (optional, for added sweetness)

Instructions:

1. Place all ingredients in a blender.
2. Blend until smooth and creamy.
3. Taste and add honey or maple syrup if desired for sweetness.
4. Pour into glasses and enjoy immediately.

Nutritional Information (per serving):

- Calories: 180
- Protein: 5g
- Fat: 8g
- Carbohydrates: 25g
- Fiber: 4g
- Sugars: 15g

2. Pineapple Coconut Green Dream

Ingredients:

- 1/2 cup pineapple chunks (fresh or frozen)
- 1/2 ripe banana
- 1/2 cup spinach leaves
- 1/2 cup coconut water
- 1/4 avocado
- Juice of 1/2 lime

Instructions:

1. Add all ingredients to a blender.
2. Blend until smooth and creamy.
3. Pour into glasses and garnish with a slice of lime if desired.

Nutritional Information (per serving):

- Calories: 160
- Protein: 3g
- Fat: 7g / Carbohydrates: 25g
- Fiber: 5g / Sugars: 15g

3. Creamy Coconut Pineapple Protein Powerhouse

Ingredients:

- 1/2 cup pineapple chunks (fresh or frozen)
- 1/2 ripe banana
- 1/2 cup spinach leaves
- 1/2 cup coconut milk
- 1 scoop vanilla protein powder
- 1 tablespoon almond butter

Instructions:

1. Combine all ingredients in a blender.
2. Blend until smooth and creamy.
3. Pour into glasses and serve chilled.

Nutritional Information (per serving):

- Calories: 250
- Protein: 20g
- Fat: 10g
- Carbohydrates: 25g
- Fiber: 4g
- Sugars: 15g

4. Pineapple Coconut Chia Paradise

Ingredients:

- 1/2 cup pineapple chunks (fresh or frozen)
- 1/2 ripe banana
- 1/2 cup spinach leaves
- 1/2 cup coconut water

- 1 tablespoon chia seeds

- 1 teaspoon honey or maple syrup (optional, for added sweetness)

Instructions:

1. Add all ingredients to a blender.

2. Blend until smooth and creamy.

3. Taste and add honey or maple syrup if desired.

4. Pour into glasses and top with additional chia seeds for added texture.

Nutritional Information (per serving):

- Calories: 190

- Protein: 4g

- Fat: 8g

- Carbohydrates: 30g

- Fiber: 7g

- Sugars: 15g

5. Pineapple Coconut Ginger Zing

Ingredients:

- 1/2 cup pineapple chunks (fresh or frozen)

- 1/2 ripe banana

- 1/2 cup spinach leaves

- 1/2 cup coconut milk

- 1 teaspoon grated ginger

- 1/4 teaspoon ground turmeric

Instructions:

1. Place all ingredients in a blender.

2. Blend until smooth and creamy.

3. Pour into glasses and serve chilled.

Nutritional Information (per serving):

- Calories: 200

- Protein: 4g

- Fat: 8g

- Carbohydrates: 30g

- Fiber: 5g

- Sugars: 15g

These Creamy Coconut Pineapple smoothie variations offer a tropical and refreshing way to support digestive health and manage hiatal hernia symptoms. Packed with nutrient-rich ingredients and tropical flavors, these smoothies provide a delicious and soothing option for individuals seeking digestive comfort and overall well-being. Enjoy these creamy delights as a nourishing breakfast, post-workout refresher, or afternoon snack, and feel confident knowing you're giving your body the care and nourishment it deserves.

Healing Turmeric Mango: Anti-Inflammatory Elixir to Calm Digestive Discomfort

As a registered dietitian specializing in digestive health, I've developed these Healing Turmeric Mango smoothie variations to offer a soothing and anti-inflammatory option for individuals managing hiatal hernia symptoms. Packed with healing ingredients like turmeric and mango, these smoothies are designed to calm digestive discomfort and promote overall well-being. Enjoy these nutritious elixirs any time of day for a refreshing boost of nutrients.

1. Classic Turmeric Mango Blend

Ingredients:

- 1/2 cup frozen mango chunks
- 1/2 ripe banana
- 1/2 cup spinach leaves
- 1/2 cup almond milk (or dairy-free milk of choice)
- 1 teaspoon grated fresh turmeric (or 1/2 teaspoon ground turmeric)
- 1 tablespoon honey or maple syrup (optional, for added sweetness)

Instructions:

1. Place all ingredients in a blender.
2. Blend until smooth and creamy.
3. Taste and add honey or maple syrup if desired for sweetness.
4. Pour into glasses and enjoy immediately.

Nutritional Information (per serving):

- Calories: 160

- Protein: 3g

- Fat: 2g

- Carbohydrates: 35g

- Fiber: 5g

- Sugars: 25g

2. Turmeric Mango Coconut Dream

Ingredients:

- 1/2 cup frozen mango chunks

- 1/2 ripe banana

- 1/2 cup spinach leaves

- 1/2 cup coconut water

- 1 tablespoon shredded coconut

- 1/2 teaspoon grated fresh turmeric (or 1/4 teaspoon ground turmeric)

Instructions:

1. Add all ingredients to a blender.

2. Blend until smooth and creamy.

3. Pour into glasses and garnish with a sprinkle of shredded coconut.

Nutritional Information (per serving):

- Calories: 140

- Protein: 2g

- Fat: 3g

- Carbohydrates: 30g

- Fiber: 5g

- Sugars: 20g

3. Mango Turmeric Ginger Zinger

Ingredients:

- 1/2 cup frozen mango chunks

- 1/2 ripe banana

- 1/2 cup spinach leaves

- 1/2 cup almond milk (or dairy-free milk of choice)

- 1 teaspoon grated fresh turmeric (or 1/2 teaspoon ground turmeric)

- 1 teaspoon grated fresh ginger

Instructions:

1. Combine all ingredients in a blender.

2. Blend until smooth and creamy.

3. Pour into glasses and serve chilled.

Nutritional Information (per serving):

- Calories: 150

- Protein: 3g

- Fat: 2g

- Carbohydrates: 35g

- Fiber: 5g

- Sugars: 20g

4. Turmeric Mango Pineapple Paradise

Ingredients:

- 1/2 cup frozen mango chunks
- 1/2 cup frozen pineapple chunks
- 1/2 ripe banana
- 1/2 cup spinach leaves
- 1/2 cup coconut water
- 1/2 teaspoon grated fresh turmeric (or 1/4 teaspoon ground turmeric)

Instructions:

1. Place all ingredients in a blender.
2. Blend until smooth and creamy.
3. Pour into glasses and garnish with a pineapple slice if desired.

Nutritional Information (per serving):

- Calories: 160
- Protein: 3g
- Fat: 1g
- Carbohydrates: 35g
- Fiber: 5g
- Sugars: 25g

5. Turmeric Mango Protein Powerhouse

Ingredients:

- 1/2 cup frozen mango chunks
- 1/2 ripe banana
- 1/2 cup spinach leaves
- 1/2 cup Greek yogurt (or dairy-free yogurt)
- 1 tablespoon almond butter
- 1 teaspoon grated fresh turmeric (or 1/2 teaspoon ground turmeric)

Instructions:

1. Add all ingredients to a blender.
2. Blend until smooth and creamy.
3. Pour into glasses and top with a sprinkle of ground turmeric for garnish.

Nutritional Information (per serving):

- Calories: 250
- Protein: 15g
- Fat: 8g
- Carbohydrates: 35g
- Fiber: 5g
- Sugars: 20g

These Healing Turmeric Mango smoothie variations offer a delicious and nutritious way to calm digestive discomfort and support overall well-being. Packed with anti-inflammatory ingredients like turmeric and mango, these smoothies provide a soothing elixir for individuals managing hiatal hernia symptoms. Enjoy the vibrant flavors and healing properties of these smoothies as part of your daily routine.

Soothing Oatmeal Spice: Nourishing and Comforting Smoothie for Hiatal Hernia Relief

As a registered dietitian specializing in digestive health, I've crafted these Soothing Oatmeal Spice smoothie variations to provide a nourishing and comforting option for individuals seeking relief from hiatal hernia symptoms. Packed with soothing ingredients like oats and warming spices, these smoothies are designed to calm digestive discomfort and promote overall well-being. Enjoy these nourishing blends any time of day for a comforting boost of nutrients.

1. Classic Oatmeal Spice Blend

Ingredients:

- 1/2 cup cooked oatmeal (cooled)
- 1/2 ripe banana
- 1/2 cup almond milk (or dairy-free milk of choice)
- 1/2 teaspoon ground cinnamon
- 1/4 teaspoon ground ginger
- 1 tablespoon honey or maple syrup (optional, for added sweetness)

Instructions:

1. Place all ingredients in a blender.
2. Blend until smooth and creamy.
3. Taste and add honey or maple syrup if desired for sweetness.
4. Pour into glasses and enjoy immediately.

Nutritional Information (per serving):

- Calories: 200
- Protein: 5g
- Fat: 3g
- Carbohydrates: 40g
- Fiber: 6g
- Sugars: 15g

2. Oatmeal Spice Pumpkin Pie Delight

Ingredients:

- 1/2 cup cooked oatmeal (cooled)
- 1/2 ripe banana
- 1/4 cup pumpkin puree
- 1/2 cup almond milk (or dairy-free milk of choice)
- 1/2 teaspoon ground cinnamon
- 1/4 teaspoon ground nutmeg
- 1 tablespoon honey or maple syrup (optional, for added sweetness)

Instructions:

1. Add all ingredients to a blender.
2. Blend until smooth and creamy.
3. Pour into glasses and sprinkle with a dash of cinnamon for garnish.

Nutritional Information (per serving):

- Calories: 220
- Protein: 5g

- Fat: 3g

- Carbohydrates: 45g

- Fiber: 7g

- Sugars: 20g

3. Oatmeal Spice Apple Cinnamon Bliss

Ingredients:

- 1/2 cup cooked oatmeal (cooled)

- 1/2 ripe banana

- 1/2 cup unsweetened applesauce

- 1/2 cup almond milk (or dairy-free milk of choice)

- 1/2 teaspoon ground cinnamon

- 1/4 teaspoon ground nutmeg

- 1 tablespoon honey or maple syrup (optional, for added sweetness)

Instructions:

1. Combine all ingredients in a blender.

2. Blend until smooth and creamy.

3. Pour into glasses and garnish with a cinnamon stick for a festive touch.

Nutritional Information (per serving):

- Calories: 210

- Protein: 5g

- Fat: 3g

- Carbohydrates: 45g

- Fiber: 6g

- Sugars: 20g

4. Oatmeal Spice Chai Latte Smoothie

Ingredients:

- 1/2 cup cooked oatmeal (cooled)
- 1/2 ripe banana
- 1/2 cup brewed chai tea (cooled)
- 1/2 cup almond milk (or dairy-free milk of choice)
- 1/2 teaspoon ground cinnamon
- 1/4 teaspoon ground cardamom
- 1 tablespoon honey or maple syrup (optional, for added sweetness)

Instructions:

1. Add all ingredients to a blender.
2. Blend until smooth and creamy.
3. Pour into glasses and sprinkle with a pinch of ground cinnamon for garnish.

Nutritional Information (per serving):

- Calories: 210
- Protein: 5g
- Fat: 3g
- Carbohydrates: 45g
- Fiber: 6g
- Sugars: 20g

5. Oatmeal Spice Gingerbread Smoothie

Ingredients:

- 1/2 cup cooked oatmeal (cooled)
- 1/2 ripe banana
- 1/2 cup almond milk (or dairy-free milk of choice)
- 1/2 teaspoon ground cinnamon
- 1/4 teaspoon ground ginger
- 1/4 teaspoon ground cloves
- 1 tablespoon molasses (optional, for added sweetness)

Instructions:

1. Place all ingredients in a blender.
2. Blend until smooth and creamy.
3. Taste and add molasses if desired for sweetness.
4. Pour into glasses and sprinkle with a dash of cinnamon for garnish.

Nutritional Information (per serving):

- Calories: 220
- Protein: 5g
- Fat: 3g
- Carbohydrates: 45g
- Fiber: 6g
- Sugars: 20g

These Soothing Oatmeal Spice smoothie variations offer a comforting and nourishing way to alleviate hiatal hernia symptoms and promote overall well-being. Enjoy the warming flavors of oats and spices in each sip, knowing you're giving your body the care and nourishment it deserves. Incorporate these comforting smoothies into your daily routine for a soothing boost of nutrients and digestive relief.

Cooling Cucumber Mint: Refreshing Blend to Soothe Digestive Discomfort

As a registered dietitian specializing in digestive health, I've created these Cooling Cucumber Mint smoothie variations to offer a refreshing and soothing option for individuals seeking relief from hiatal hernia symptoms. Packed with hydrating cucumber and calming mint, these smoothies are designed to ease digestive discomfort and promote overall well-being. Enjoy these revitalizing blends any time of day for a refreshing boost of nutrients.

1. Classic Cucumber Mint Blend

Ingredients:

- 1/2 cucumber, peeled and chopped
- Handful of fresh mint leaves
- 1/2 cup spinach leaves
- 1/2 ripe banana
- 1/2 cup coconut water
- Juice of 1/2 lime

Instructions:

1. Place all ingredients in a blender.
2. Blend until smooth and creamy.
3. Pour into glasses and garnish with a mint sprig.

Nutritional Information (per serving):

- Calories: 70
- Protein: 2g
- Fat: 0g

- Carbohydrates: 15g

- Fiber: 3g

- Sugars: 7g

2. Cucumber Mint Pineapple Refresher

Ingredients:

- 1/2 cucumber, peeled and chopped

- Handful of fresh mint leaves

- 1/2 cup frozen pineapple chunks

- 1/2 cup spinach leaves

- 1/2 cup coconut water

Instructions:

1. Add all ingredients to a blender.

2. Blend until smooth and creamy.

3. Pour into glasses and enjoy immediately.

Nutritional Information (per serving):

- Calories: 90

- Protein: 2g

- Fat: 0g

- Carbohydrates: 20g

- Fiber: 4g

- Sugars: 12g

3. Cucumber Mint Yogurt Delight

Ingredients:

- 1/2 cucumber, peeled and chopped
- Handful of fresh mint leaves
- 1/2 cup Greek yogurt (or dairy-free yogurt)
- 1/2 ripe banana
- 1/2 cup almond milk (or dairy-free milk of choice)

Instructions:

1. Combine all ingredients in a blender.
2. Blend until smooth and creamy.
3. Pour into glasses and serve chilled.

Nutritional Information (per serving):

- Calories: 100
- Protein: 6g
- Fat: 2g
- Carbohydrates: 20g
- Fiber: 3g
- Sugars: 10g

4. Cucumber Mint Ginger Cooler

Ingredients:

- 1/2 cucumber, peeled and chopped
- Handful of fresh mint leaves
- 1/2 inch piece of fresh ginger, peeled
- 1/2 cup spinach leaves
- 1/2 ripe banana

- 1/2 cup coconut water

Instructions:

1. Place all ingredients in a blender.
2. Blend until smooth and creamy.
3. Pour into glasses and garnish with a cucumber slice.

Nutritional Information (per serving):

- Calories: 80
- Protein: 2g
- Fat: 0g
- Carbohydrates: 18g
- Fiber: 3g
- Sugars: 8g

5. Cucumber Mint Lemonade Smoothie

Ingredients:

- 1/2 cucumber, peeled and chopped
- Handful of fresh mint leaves
- Juice of 1 lemon
- Zest of 1 lemon
- 1/2 ripe banana
- 1/2 cup coconut water

Instructions:

1. Add all ingredients to a blender.
2. Blend until smooth and creamy.
3. Pour into glasses and garnish with a lemon slice.

Nutritional Information (per serving):

- Calories: 80

- Protein: 2g

- Fat: 0g

- Carbohydrates: 20g

- Fiber: 4g

- Sugars: 10g

These Cooling Cucumber Mint smoothie variations offer a refreshing and soothing way to alleviate hiatal hernia symptoms and promote overall well-being. Enjoy the hydrating blend of cucumber and the calming essence of mint in each sip, knowing you're giving your body the care and nourishment it deserves. Incorporate these revitalizing smoothies into your daily routine for a refreshing boost of nutrients and digestive relief.

Peachy Keen Almond: Creamy and Nutty Smoothie for Gentle Digestion

As a registered dietitian specializing in digestive health, I've crafted these Peachy Keen Almond smoothie variations to provide a creamy and nutty option for individuals seeking relief from hiatal hernia symptoms. Packed with gentle ingredients like peaches and almonds, these smoothies are designed to support gentle digestion and promote overall well-being. Enjoy these delightful blends any time of day for a nourishing boost of nutrients.

1. Classic Peachy Almond Blend

Ingredients:

- 1 ripe peach, pitted and chopped
- 1/4 cup almond butter
- 1/2 cup Greek yogurt (or dairy-free yogurt)
- 1/2 cup almond milk (or dairy-free milk of choice)
- 1 tablespoon honey or maple syrup (optional, for added sweetness)
- Handful of ice cubes

Instructions:

1. Place all ingredients in a blender.
2. Blend until smooth and creamy.
3. Taste and add honey or maple syrup if desired for sweetness.
4. Pour into glasses and serve chilled.

Nutritional Information (per serving):

- Calories: 250

- Protein: 10g

- Fat: 15g

- Carbohydrates: 25g

- Fiber: 5g

- Sugars: 18g

2. Peach Almond Spinach Delight

Ingredients:

- 1 ripe peach, pitted and chopped

- 1/4 cup almond butter

- 1/2 cup spinach leaves

- 1/2 cup almond milk (or dairy-free milk of choice)

- 1/2 ripe banana

- Handful of ice cubes

Instructions:

1. Add all ingredients to a blender.

2. Blend until smooth and creamy.

3. Pour into glasses and garnish with a peach slice.

Nutritional Information (per serving):

- Calories: 230

- Protein: 9g

- Fat: 14g

- Carbohydrates: 25g

- Fiber: 6g

- Sugars: 17g

3. Peach Almond Coconut Dream

Ingredients:

- 1 ripe peach, pitted and chopped
- 1/4 cup almond butter
- 1/2 cup coconut milk
- 1/2 cup Greek yogurt (or dairy-free yogurt)
- Handful of ice cubes

Instructions:

1. Combine all ingredients in a blender.
2. Blend until smooth and creamy.
3. Pour into glasses and serve chilled.

Nutritional Information (per serving):

- Calories: 270
- Protein: 11g
- Fat: 16g
- Carbohydrates: 26g
- Fiber: 5g
- Sugars: 20g

4. Peachy Almond Vanilla Bean Smoothie

Ingredients:

- 1 ripe peach, pitted and chopped
- 1/4 cup almond butter
- 1/2 cup almond milk (or dairy-free milk of choice)
- 1/2 cup Greek yogurt (or dairy-free yogurt)

- 1 teaspoon vanilla extract
- Handful of ice cubes

Instructions:

1. Place all ingredients in a blender.
2. Blend until smooth and creamy.
3. Pour into glasses and garnish with a sprinkle of cinnamon.

Nutritional Information (per serving):

- Calories: 240
- Protein: 10g
- Fat: 14g
- Carbohydrates: 24g
- Fiber: 4g
- Sugars: 16g

5. Peachy Almond Green Power Smoothie

Ingredients:

- 1 ripe peach, pitted and chopped
- 1/4 cup almond butter
- 1/2 cup spinach leaves
- 1/2 cup almond milk (or dairy-free milk of choice)
- 1/2 ripe banana
- Handful of ice cubes

Instructions:

1. Add all ingredients to a blender.
2. Blend until smooth and creamy.

3. Pour into glasses and garnish with a peach slice.

Nutritional Information (per serving):

- Calories: 240

- Protein: 10g

- Fat: 14g

- Carbohydrates: 25g

- Fiber: 6g

- Sugars: 18g

These Peachy Keen Almond smoothie variations offer a creamy and nutty option for individuals seeking relief from hiatal hernia symptoms. Packed with gentle ingredients like peaches and almonds, these smoothies provide a nourishing and delicious option for supporting gentle digestion and promoting overall well-being. Enjoy these delightful blends as part of your daily routine for a delicious and comforting boost of nutrients.

Zesty Carrot Ginger: Energizing Blend with A Hint of Spice for Digestive Relief

As a registered dietitian specializing in digestive health, I've curated these Zesty Carrot Ginger smoothie variations to provide an energizing and digestive relief option for individuals managing hiatal hernia symptoms. Packed with nutrient-rich carrots and invigorating ginger, these smoothies are designed to support digestion and promote overall well-being. Enjoy these vibrant blends any time of day for a refreshing boost of nutrients.

1. Classic Carrot Ginger Blend

Ingredients:

- 1 medium carrot, peeled and chopped
- 1/2 inch piece of fresh ginger, peeled
- 1/2 ripe banana
- 1/2 cup Greek yogurt (or dairy-free yogurt)
- 1/2 cup almond milk (or dairy-free milk of choice)
- Juice of 1/2 lemon
- Handful of ice cubes

Instructions:

1. Place all ingredients in a blender.
2. Blend until smooth and creamy.
3. Pour into glasses and serve chilled.

Nutritional Information (per serving):

- Calories: 120
- Protein: 6g

- Fat: 2g

- Carbohydrates: 20g

- Fiber: 4g

- Sugars: 12g

2. Carrot Ginger Orange Sunrise

Ingredients:

- 1 medium carrot, peeled and chopped

- 1/2 inch piece of fresh ginger, peeled

- 1/2 ripe banana

- 1/2 cup orange juice

- 1/2 cup Greek yogurt (or dairy-free yogurt)

- Handful of ice cubes

Instructions:

1. Add all ingredients to a blender.

2. Blend until smooth and creamy.

3. Pour into glasses and garnish with an orange slice.

Nutritional Information (per serving):

- Calories: 140

- Protein: 5g

- Fat: 2g

- Carbohydrates: 25g

- Fiber: 4g

- Sugars: 15g

3. Carrot Ginger Pineapple Punch

Ingredients:

- 1 medium carrot, peeled and chopped
- 1/2 inch piece of fresh ginger, peeled
- 1/2 cup chopped pineapple
- 1/2 ripe banana
- 1/2 cup coconut water
- Handful of ice cubes

Instructions:

1. Combine all ingredients in a blender.
2. Blend until smooth and creamy.
3. Pour into glasses and garnish with a pineapple wedge.

Nutritional Information (per serving):

- Calories: 130
- Protein: 4g
- Fat: 1g
- Carbohydrates: 30g
- Fiber: 5g
- Sugars: 18g

4. Carrot Ginger Green Power Smoothie

Ingredients:

- 1 medium carrot, peeled and chopped
- 1/2 inch piece of fresh ginger, peeled
- 1/2 cup spinach leaves

- 1/2 ripe banana
- 1/2 cup almond milk (or dairy-free milk of choice)
- Handful of ice cubes

Instructions:

1. Place all ingredients in a blender.
2. Blend until smooth and creamy.
3. Pour into glasses and enjoy immediately.

Nutritional Information (per serving):

- Calories: 110
- Protein: 4g
- Fat: 1g
- Carbohydrates: 25g
- Fiber: 5g
- Sugars: 15g

5. Carrot Ginger Turmeric Elixir

Ingredients:

- 1 medium carrot, peeled and chopped
- 1/2 inch piece of fresh ginger, peeled
- 1/2 teaspoon ground turmeric
- 1/2 ripe banana
- 1/2 cup almond milk (or dairy-free milk of choice)
- 1 tablespoon honey or maple syrup (optional, for added sweetness)
- Handful of ice cubes

Instructions:

1. Add all ingredients to a blender.
2. Blend until smooth and creamy.
3. Taste and add honey or maple syrup if desired for sweetness.
4. Pour into glasses and serve chilled.

Nutritional Information (per serving):

- Calories: 130
- Protein: 4g
- Fat: 2g
- Carbohydrates: 30g
- Fiber: 5g
- Sugars: 18g

These Zesty Carrot Ginger smoothie variations offer an energizing and digestive relief option for individuals managing hiatal hernia symptoms. Packed with nutrient-rich ingredients like carrots and ginger, these smoothies provide a refreshing and nourishing way to support digestion and promote overall well-being. Incorporate these vibrant blends into your daily routine for a delicious and invigorating boost of nutrients.

Spinach Avocado Dream: Creamy Green Smoothie Packed with Nutrients and Fiber

As a registered dietitian specializing in digestive health, I've crafted these Spinach Avocado Dream smoothie variations to offer a creamy and nutrient-packed option for individuals managing hiatal hernia symptoms. Loaded with fiber-rich spinach and healthy fats from avocado, these smoothies are designed to support digestive health and promote overall well-being. Enjoy these nourishing blends any time of day for a delicious boost of nutrients.

1. Classic Spinach Avocado Blend

Ingredients:

- 1 cup fresh spinach leaves
- 1/2 ripe avocado
- 1/2 banana
- 1/2 cup Greek yogurt (or dairy-free yogurt)
- 1/2 cup almond milk (or dairy-free milk of choice)
- Handful of ice cubes

Instructions:

1. Place all ingredients in a blender.
2. Blend until smooth and creamy.
3. Pour into glasses and enjoy immediately.

Nutritional Information (per serving):

- Calories: 180
- Protein: 7g
- Fat: 9g

- Carbohydrates: 20g

- Fiber: 6g

- Sugars: 9g

2. Spinach Avocado Berry Blast

Ingredients:

- 1 cup fresh spinach leaves

- 1/2 ripe avocado

- 1/2 cup mixed berries (such as strawberries, blueberries, and raspberries)

- 1/2 cup Greek yogurt (or dairy-free yogurt)

- 1/2 cup almond milk (or dairy-free milk of choice)

- Handful of ice cubes

Instructions:

1. Add all ingredients to a blender.

2. Blend until smooth and creamy.

3. Pour into glasses and garnish with a few fresh berries.

Nutritional Information (per serving):

- Calories: 200

- Protein: 7g

- Fat: 9g

- Carbohydrates: 25g

- Fiber: 8g

- Sugars: 13g

3. Spinach Avocado Mango Magic

Ingredients:

- 1 cup fresh spinach leaves
- 1/2 ripe avocado
- 1/2 cup chopped mango
- 1/2 cup Greek yogurt (or dairy-free yogurt)
- 1/2 cup coconut water
- Handful of ice cubes

Instructions:

1. Combine all ingredients in a blender.
2. Blend until smooth and creamy.
3. Pour into glasses and garnish with a mango slice.

Nutritional Information (per serving):

- Calories: 190
- Protein: 7g
- Fat: 9g
- Carbohydrates: 25g
- Fiber: 7g
- Sugars: 15g

4. Spinach Avocado Banana Smoothie

Ingredients:

- 1 cup fresh spinach leaves
- 1/2 ripe avocado
- 1/2 banana
- 1/2 cup almond milk (or dairy-free milk of choice)

- 1 tablespoon honey or maple syrup (optional, for added sweetness)
- Handful of ice cubes

Instructions:

1. Place all ingredients in a blender.
2. Blend until smooth and creamy.
3. Taste and add honey or maple syrup if desired for sweetness.
4. Pour into glasses and serve chilled.

Nutritional Information (per serving):

- Calories: 190
- Protein: 6g
- Fat: 9g
- Carbohydrates: 25g
- Fiber: 6g
- Sugars: 14g

5. Spinach Avocado Protein Powerhouse

Ingredients:

- 1 cup fresh spinach leaves
- 1/2 ripe avocado
- 1/2 cup Greek yogurt (or dairy-free yogurt)
- 1/2 cup almond milk (or dairy-free milk of choice)
- 1 scoop protein powder (vanilla or unflavored)
- Handful of ice cubes

Instructions:

1. Add all ingredients to a blender.

2. Blend until smooth and creamy.

3. Pour into glasses and enjoy immediately.

Nutritional Information (per serving):

- Calories: 250

- Protein: 20g

- Fat: 12g

- Carbohydrates: 15g

- Fiber: 5g

- Sugars: 7g

These Spinach Avocado Dream smoothie variations offer a creamy and nutrient-packed option for individuals managing hiatal hernia symptoms. Loaded with fiber-rich spinach and healthy fats from avocado, these smoothies provide a delicious and nourishing way to support digestive health and promote overall well-being. Incorporate these nutrient-rich blends into your daily routine for a refreshing boost of nutrients and fiber.

Vanilla Banana Chai: Comforting and Fragrant Smoothie to Calm Hiatal Hernia Symptoms

As a registered dietitian specializing in digestive health, I've created these Vanilla Banana Chai smoothie variations to offer a comforting and fragrant option for individuals seeking relief from hiatal hernia symptoms. Infused with the soothing flavors of vanilla and chai spices, these smoothies are designed to calm digestive discomfort and promote overall well-being. Enjoy these aromatic blends any time of day for a comforting boost of nutrients.

1. Classic Vanilla Banana Chai Blend

Ingredients:

- 1 ripe banana
- 1/2 teaspoon vanilla extract
- 1/2 teaspoon ground cinnamon
- 1/4 teaspoon ground ginger
- Pinch of ground cloves
- Pinch of ground nutmeg
- 1/2 cup Greek yogurt (or dairy-free yogurt)
- 1/2 cup almond milk (or dairy-free milk of choice)
- Handful of ice cubes

Instructions:

1. Place all ingredients in a blender.
2. Blend until smooth and creamy.
3. Pour into glasses and serve chilled.

Nutritional Information (per serving):

- Calories: 160
- Protein: 6g
- Fat: 1g
- Carbohydrates: 30g
- Fiber: 4g
- Sugars: 16g

2. Vanilla Banana Chai Protein Power

Ingredients:

- 1 ripe banana
- 1/2 teaspoon vanilla extract
- 1/2 teaspoon ground cinnamon
- 1/4 teaspoon ground ginger
- Pinch of ground cloves
- Pinch of ground nutmeg
- 1/2 cup Greek yogurt (or dairy-free yogurt)
- 1/2 cup almond milk (or dairy-free milk of choice)
- 1 scoop vanilla protein powder
- Handful of ice cubes

Instructions:

1. Add all ingredients to a blender.
2. Blend until smooth and creamy.
3. Pour into glasses and enjoy immediately.

Nutritional Information (per serving):

- Calories: 220
- Protein: 20g
- Fat: 2g
- Carbohydrates: 30g
- Fiber: 5g
- Sugars: 18g

3. Vanilla Banana Chai Coconut Delight

Ingredients:

- 1 ripe banana
- 1/2 teaspoon vanilla extract
- 1/2 teaspoon ground cinnamon
- 1/4 teaspoon ground ginger
- Pinch of ground cloves
- Pinch of ground nutmeg
- 1/2 cup coconut milk
- 1/2 cup Greek yogurt (or dairy-free yogurt)
- Handful of ice cubes

Instructions:

1. Combine all ingredients in a blender.
2. Blend until smooth and creamy.
3. Pour into glasses and garnish with a sprinkle of cinnamon.

Nutritional Information (per serving):

- Calories: 180
- Protein: 7g
- Fat: 5g
- Carbohydrates: 30g
- Fiber: 4g
- Sugars: 16g

4. Vanilla Banana Chai Oatmeal Smoothie

Ingredients:

- 1 ripe banana
- 1/2 teaspoon vanilla extract
- 1/2 teaspoon ground cinnamon
- 1/4 teaspoon ground ginger
- Pinch of ground cloves
- Pinch of ground nutmeg
- 1/4 cup rolled oats
- 1/2 cup Greek yogurt (or dairy-free yogurt)
- 1/2 cup almond milk (or dairy-free milk of choice)
- Handful of ice cubes

Instructions:

1. Place all ingredients in a blender.
2. Blend until smooth and creamy.
3. Pour into glasses and serve chilled.

Nutritional Information (per serving):

- Calories: 200
- Protein: 8g
- Fat: 2g
- Carbohydrates: 35g
- Fiber: 5g
- Sugars: 16g

5. Vanilla Banana Chai Green Power Smoothie

Ingredients:

- 1 ripe banana
- 1/2 teaspoon vanilla extract
- 1/2 teaspoon ground cinnamon
- 1/4 teaspoon ground ginger
- Pinch of ground cloves
- Pinch of ground nutmeg
- 1 cup fresh spinach leaves
- 1/2 cup Greek yogurt (or dairy-free yogurt)
- 1/2 cup almond milk (or dairy-free milk of choice)
- Handful of ice cubes

Instructions:

1. Add all ingredients to a blender.
2. Blend until smooth and creamy.
3. Pour into glasses and enjoy immediately.

Nutritional Information (per serving):

- Calories: 170

- Protein: 8g

- Fat: 2g

- Carbohydrates: 30g

- Fiber: 6g

- Sugars: 16g

These Vanilla Banana Chai smoothie variations offer a comforting and fragrant option for individuals seeking relief from hiatal hernia symptoms. Infused with the soothing flavors of vanilla and chai spices, these smoothies provide a delicious and calming way to support digestive health and promote overall well-being. Incorporate these aromatic blends into your daily routine for a comforting boost of nutrients and flavor.

Blueberry Basil Bliss: Antioxidant-Rich Mix with A Refreshing Twist For Digestive Support

As a registered dietitian specializing in digestive health, I've curated these Blueberry Basil Bliss smoothie variations to offer an antioxidant-rich mix with a refreshing twist for individuals seeking digestive support, especially those managing hiatal hernia symptoms. Packed with nutrient-dense blueberries and aromatic basil, these smoothies are designed to soothe the digestive system and promote overall well-being. Enjoy these refreshing blends any time of day for a burst of flavor and nourishment.

1. Classic Blueberry Basil Blend

Ingredients:

- 1 cup fresh or frozen blueberries
- Handful of fresh basil leaves
- 1/2 cup Greek yogurt (or dairy-free yogurt)
- 1/2 cup almond milk (or dairy-free milk of choice)
- 1 tablespoon honey or maple syrup (optional, for added sweetness)
- Handful of ice cubes

Instructions:

1. Place all ingredients in a blender.
2. Blend until smooth and creamy.
3. Taste and add honey or maple syrup if desired for sweetness.
4. Pour into glasses and serve chilled.

Nutritional Information (per serving):

- Calories: 150
- Protein: 6g
- Fat: 2g
- Carbohydrates: 25g
- Fiber: 5g
- Sugars: 18g

2. Blueberry Basil Green Power Smoothie

Ingredients:

- 1 cup fresh or frozen blueberries
- Handful of fresh basil leaves
- 1/2 cup spinach leaves
- 1/2 ripe banana
- 1/2 cup almond milk (or dairy-free milk of choice)
- Handful of ice cubes

Instructions:

1. Add all ingredients to a blender.
2. Blend until smooth and creamy.
3. Pour into glasses and garnish with a basil leaf.

Nutritional Information (per serving):

- Calories: 160
- Protein: 6g
- Fat: 2g
- Carbohydrates: 30g
- Fiber: 6g

- Sugars: 18g

3. Blueberry Basil Coconut Cooler

Ingredients:

- 1 cup fresh or frozen blueberries
- Handful of fresh basil leaves
- 1/2 cup coconut water
- 1/2 cup Greek yogurt (or dairy-free yogurt)
- Handful of ice cubes

Instructions:

1. Combine all ingredients in a blender.
2. Blend until smooth and creamy.
3. Pour into glasses and garnish with a sprinkle of shredded coconut.

Nutritional Information (per serving):

- Calories: 140
- Protein: 6g
- Fat: 2g
- Carbohydrates: 25g
- Fiber: 5g
- Sugars: 15g

4. Blueberry Basil Pineapple Paradise

Ingredients:

- 1 cup fresh or frozen blueberries
- Handful of fresh basil leaves
- 1/2 cup chopped pineapple
- 1/2 cup Greek yogurt (or dairy-free yogurt)
- 1/2 cup almond milk (or dairy-free milk of choice)
- Handful of ice cubes

Instructions:

1. Place all ingredients in a blender.
2. Blend until smooth and creamy.
3. Pour into glasses and garnish with a pineapple wedge.

Nutritional Information (per serving):

- Calories: 160
- Protein: 6g
- Fat: 2g
- Carbohydrates: 30g
- Fiber: 6g
- Sugars: 20g

5. Blueberry Basil Mango Tango

Ingredients:

- 1 cup fresh or frozen blueberries
- Handful of fresh basil leaves
- 1/2 cup chopped mango

- 1/2 cup Greek yogurt (or dairy-free yogurt)

- 1/2 cup almond milk (or dairy-free milk of choice)

- Handful of ice cubes

Instructions:

1. Add all ingredients to a blender.

2. Blend until smooth and creamy.

3. Pour into glasses and garnish with a basil leaf.

Nutritional Information (per serving):

- Calories: 170

- Protein: 6g

- Fat: 2g

- Carbohydrates: 30g

- Fiber: 6g

- Sugars: 20g

These Blueberry Basil Bliss smoothie variations offer an antioxidant-rich mix with a refreshing twist for individuals seeking digestive support, especially those managing hiatal hernia symptoms. Packed with nutrient-dense blueberries and aromatic basil, these smoothies provide a flavorful and nourishing way to support digestive health and promote overall well-being. Incorporate these refreshing blends into your daily routine for a delicious and revitalizing boost of nutrients and flavor.

Pumpkin Spice Protein: Warm and Filling Smoothie for Sustained Energy and Digestive Comfort

As a registered dietitian specializing in digestive health, I've developed these Pumpkin Spice Protein smoothie variations to offer a warm and filling option for individuals seeking sustained energy and digestive comfort, particularly those managing hiatal hernia symptoms. Infused with the cozy flavors of pumpkin spice, these smoothies are packed with protein and fiber to support digestive health and promote overall well-being. Enjoy these comforting blends any time of day for a nourishing and satisfying treat.

1. Classic Pumpkin Spice Protein Blend

Ingredients:

- 1/2 cup canned pumpkin puree
- 1/2 ripe banana
- 1 scoop vanilla protein powder
- 1/2 teaspoon pumpkin pie spice
- 1/2 cup Greek yogurt (or dairy-free yogurt)
- 1/2 cup almond milk (or dairy-free milk of choice)
- Handful of ice cubes

Instructions:

1. Place all ingredients in a blender.
2. Blend until smooth and creamy.
3. Pour into a microwave-safe mug and heat in the microwave for 1-2 minutes until warm.
4. Stir well before enjoying.

Nutritional Information (per serving):

- Calories: 220
- Protein: 20g
- Fat: 3g
- Carbohydrates: 30g
- Fiber: 6g
- Sugars: 15g

2. Pumpkin Spice Protein Oatmeal Smoothie

Ingredients:

- 1/2 cup canned pumpkin puree
- 1/2 ripe banana
- 1 scoop vanilla protein powder
- 1/2 teaspoon pumpkin pie spice
- 1/4 cup rolled oats
- 1/2 cup Greek yogurt (or dairy-free yogurt)
- 1/2 cup almond milk (or dairy-free milk of choice)
- Handful of ice cubes

Instructions:

1. Add all ingredients to a blender.
2. Blend until smooth and creamy.
3. Pour into a microwave-safe mug and heat in the microwave for 1-2 minutes until warm.
4. Stir well before enjoying.

Nutritional Information (per serving):

- Calories: 250
- Protein: 22g
- Fat: 4g
- Carbohydrates: 35g
- Fiber: 7g
- Sugars: 15g

3. Pumpkin Spice Protein Peanut Butter Delight

Ingredients:

- 1/2 cup canned pumpkin puree
- 1/2 ripe banana
- 1 scoop vanilla protein powder
- 1/2 teaspoon pumpkin pie spice
- 1 tablespoon peanut butter
- 1/2 cup Greek yogurt (or dairy-free yogurt)
- 1/2 cup almond milk (or dairy-free milk of choice)
- Handful of ice cubes

Instructions:

1. Combine all ingredients in a blender.
2. Blend until smooth and creamy.
3. Pour into a microwave-safe mug and heat in the microwave for 1-2 minutes until warm.
4. Stir well before enjoying.

Nutritional Information (per serving):

- Calories: 280
- Protein: 24g
- Fat: 9g
- Carbohydrates: 30g
- Fiber: 6g
- Sugars: 15g

4. Pumpkin Spice Protein Chia Seed Smoothie

Ingredients:

- 1/2 cup canned pumpkin puree
- 1/2 ripe banana
- 1 scoop vanilla protein powder
- 1/2 teaspoon pumpkin pie spice
- 1 tablespoon chia seeds
- 1/2 cup Greek yogurt (or dairy-free yogurt)
- 1/2 cup almond milk (or dairy-free milk of choice)
- Handful of ice cubes

Instructions:

1. Add all ingredients to a blender.
2. Blend until smooth and creamy.
3. Pour into a microwave-safe mug and heat in the microwave for 1-2 minutes until warm.
4. Stir well before enjoying.

Nutritional Information (per serving):

- Calories: 260
- Protein: 21g
- Fat: 7g
- Carbohydrates: 30g
- Fiber: 8g
- Sugars: 15g

5. Pumpkin Spice Protein Almond Smoothie

Ingredients:

- 1/2 cup canned pumpkin puree
- 1/2 ripe banana
- 1 scoop vanilla protein powder
- 1/2 teaspoon pumpkin pie spice
- 1 tablespoon almond butter
- 1/2 cup Greek yogurt (or dairy-free yogurt)
- 1/2 cup almond milk (or dairy-free milk of choice)
- Handful of ice cubes

Instructions:

1. Place all ingredients in a blender.
2. Blend until smooth and creamy.
3. Pour into a microwave-safe mug and heat in the microwave for 1-2 minutes until warm.
4. Stir well before enjoying.

Nutritional Information (per serving):

- Calories: 270
- Protein: 23g
- Fat: 8g
- Carbohydrates: 30g
- Fiber: 7g
- Sugars: 15g

These Pumpkin Spice Protein smoothie variations offer a warm and filling option for individuals seeking sustained energy and digestive comfort, especially those managing hiatal hernia symptoms. Infused with cozy pumpkin spice flavors and packed with protein and fiber, these smoothies provide a nourishing and satisfying way to support digestive health and promote overall well-being. Incorporate these comforting blends into your daily routine for a delicious and energizing treat.

Mango Coconut Cream: Tropical Indulgence with A Creamy Texture For Hiatal Hernia Relief

As a registered dietitian specializing in digestive health, I've designed these Mango Coconut Cream smoothie variations to offer a tropical indulgence with a creamy texture, ideal for individuals seeking relief from hiatal hernia symptoms. Bursting with the flavors of mango and coconut, these smoothies provide a soothing and satisfying option to support digestive comfort and overall well-being. Enjoy these luscious blends any time of day for a refreshing and nourishing treat.

1. Classic Mango Coconut Blend

Ingredients:

- 1 cup chopped mango
- 1/2 cup coconut milk
- 1/2 cup Greek yogurt (or dairy-free yogurt)
- 1 tablespoon honey or maple syrup (optional, for added sweetness)
- Handful of ice cubes

Instructions:

1. Place all ingredients in a blender.
2. Blend until smooth and creamy.
3. Taste and add honey or maple syrup if desired for sweetness.
4. Pour into glasses and serve chilled.

Nutritional Information (per serving):

- Calories: 220
- Protein: 7g
- Fat: 8g
- Carbohydrates: 30g
- Fiber: 3g
- Sugars: 25g

2. Mango Coconut Protein Power Smoothie

Ingredients:

- 1 cup chopped mango
- 1/2 cup coconut milk
- 1/2 cup Greek yogurt (or dairy-free yogurt)
- 1 scoop vanilla protein powder
- Handful of ice cubes

Instructions:

1. Add all ingredients to a blender.
2. Blend until smooth and creamy.
3. Pour into glasses and enjoy immediately.

Nutritional Information (per serving):

- Calories: 250
- Protein: 20g
- Fat: 8g
- Carbohydrates: 30g
- Fiber: 3g / Sugars: 25g

3. Mango Coconut Avocado Smoothie

Ingredients:

- 1 cup chopped mango
- 1/2 cup coconut milk
- 1/4 ripe avocado
- 1/2 cup Greek yogurt (or dairy-free yogurt)
- Handful of ice cubes

Instructions:

1. Combine all ingredients in a blender.
2. Blend until smooth and creamy.
3. Pour into glasses and garnish with a slice of mango.

Nutritional Information (per serving):

- Calories: 240
- Protein: 7g
- Fat: 9g
- Carbohydrates: 30g
- Fiber: 5g
- Sugars: 25g

4. Mango Coconut Green Goddess Smoothie

Ingredients:

- 1 cup chopped mango
- 1/2 cup coconut milk
- 1 cup spinach leaves
- 1/2 cup Greek yogurt (or dairy-free yogurt)
- Handful of ice cubes

Instructions:

1. Place all ingredients in a blender.
2. Blend until smooth and creamy.
3. Pour into glasses and serve chilled.

Nutritional Information (per serving):

- Calories: 220
- Protein: 8g
- Fat: 8g
- Carbohydrates: 30g
- Fiber: 4g
- Sugars: 25g

5. Mango Coconut Chia Bliss Smoothie

Ingredients:

- 1 cup chopped mango
- 1/2 cup coconut milk
- 1/2 cup Greek yogurt (or dairy-free yogurt)
- 1 tablespoon chia seeds
- Handful of ice cubes

Instructions:

1. Add all ingredients to a blender.
2. Blend until smooth and creamy.
3. Pour into glasses and garnish with a sprinkle of chia seeds.

Nutritional Information (per serving):

- Calories: 230

- Protein: 7g

- Fat: 9g

- Carbohydrates: 30g

- Fiber: 6g

- Sugars: 25g

These Mango Coconut Cream smoothie variations offer a tropical indulgence with a creamy texture, perfect for individuals seeking relief from hiatal hernia symptoms. Bursting with the flavors of mango and coconut, these smoothies provide a soothing and satisfying option to support digestive comfort and overall well-being. Incorporate these luscious blends into your daily routine for a refreshing and nourishing treat.

Berry Beet Boost: Vibrant and Nutrient-Dense Smoothie to Support Digestive Health

As a registered dietitian specializing in digestive health, I've crafted these Berry Beet Boost smoothie variations to offer a vibrant and nutrient-dense option for individuals seeking to support digestive health, particularly those managing hiatal hernia symptoms. Packed with the goodness of berries and beets, these smoothies provide a burst of flavor and essential nutrients to promote overall well-being. Enjoy these refreshing blends any time of day for a nourishing and satisfying treat.

1. Classic Berry Beet Blend

Ingredients:

- 1/2 cup mixed berries (such as strawberries, blueberries, and raspberries)
- 1/2 small beet, cooked and peeled
- 1/2 cup Greek yogurt (or dairy-free yogurt)
- 1/2 cup almond milk (or dairy-free milk of choice)
- 1 tablespoon honey or maple syrup (optional, for added sweetness)
- Handful of ice cubes

Instructions:

1. Place all ingredients in a blender.
2. Blend until smooth and creamy.
3. Taste and add honey or maple syrup if desired for sweetness.
4. Pour into glasses and serve chilled.

Nutritional Information (per serving):

- Calories: 180
- Protein: 7g
- Fat: 2g
- Carbohydrates: 30g
- Fiber: 5g
- Sugars: 20g

2. Berry Beet Protein Power Smoothie

Ingredients:

- 1/2 cup mixed berries (such as strawberries, blueberries, and raspberries)
- 1/2 small beet, cooked and peeled
- 1/2 cup Greek yogurt (or dairy-free yogurt)
- 1 scoop vanilla protein powder
- 1/2 cup almond milk (or dairy-free milk of choice)
- Handful of ice cubes

Instructions:

1. Add all ingredients to a blender.
2. Blend until smooth and creamy.
3. Pour into glasses and enjoy immediately.

Nutritional Information (per serving):

- Calories: 220
- Protein: 20g
- Fat: 2g
- Carbohydrates: 30g

- Fiber: 6g

- Sugars: 18g

3. Berry Beet Green Power Smoothie

Ingredients:

- 1/2 cup mixed berries (such as strawberries, blueberries, and raspberries)

- 1/2 small beet, cooked and peeled

- 1 cup spinach leaves

- 1/2 cup Greek yogurt (or dairy-free yogurt)

- 1/2 cup almond milk (or dairy-free milk of choice)

- Handful of ice cubes

Instructions:

1. Combine all ingredients in a blender.

2. Blend until smooth and creamy.

3. Pour into glasses and serve chilled.

Nutritional Information (per serving):

- Calories: 200

- Protein: 8g

- Fat: 2g

- Carbohydrates: 30g

- Fiber: 7g

- Sugars: 18g

4. Berry Beet Coconut Bliss Smoothie

Ingredients:

- 1/2 cup mixed berries (such as strawberries, blueberries, and raspberries)
- 1/2 small beet, cooked and peeled
- 1/2 cup coconut milk
- 1/2 cup Greek yogurt (or dairy-free yogurt)
- Handful of ice cubes

Instructions:

1. Place all ingredients in a blender.
2. Blend until smooth and creamy.
3. Pour into glasses and garnish with shredded coconut.

Nutritional Information (per serving):

- Calories: 190
- Protein: 7g
- Fat: 5g
- Carbohydrates: 30g
- Fiber: 6g
- Sugars: 18g

5. Berry Beet Citrus Zing Smoothie

Ingredients:

- 1/2 cup mixed berries (such as strawberries, blueberries, and raspberries)
- 1/2 small beet, cooked and peeled
- Juice of 1/2 orange

- 1/2 cup Greek yogurt (or dairy-free yogurt)

- 1/2 cup almond milk (or dairy-free milk of choice)

- Handful of ice cubes

Instructions:

1. Add all ingredients to a blender.

2. Blend until smooth and creamy.

3. Pour into glasses and garnish with a slice of orange.

Nutritional Information (per serving):

- Calories: 170

- Protein: 7g

- Fat: 2g

- Carbohydrates: 30g

- Fiber: 6g

- Sugars: 18g

These Berry Beet Boost smoothie variations offer a vibrant and nutrient-dense option for individuals seeking to support digestive health, especially those managing hiatal hernia symptoms. Packed with the goodness of berries and beets, these smoothies provide essential nutrients and a burst of flavor to promote overall well-being. Incorporate these refreshing blends into your daily routine for a nourishing and satisfying treat.

Pineapple Papaya Paradise: Tropical Fusion with Enzyme-Rich Fruits For Digestive Ease

As a registered dietitian specializing in digestive health, I've curated these Pineapple Papaya Paradise smoothie variations to offer a tropical fusion with enzyme-rich fruits, perfect for promoting digestive ease, especially for those managing hiatal hernia symptoms. Bursting with the flavors of pineapple and papaya, these smoothies are packed with enzymes that aid digestion and support overall gut health. Enjoy these refreshing blends any time of day for a delicious and soothing treat.

1. Classic Pineapple Papaya Blend

Ingredients:

- 1 cup chopped pineapple
- 1 cup chopped papaya
- 1/2 cup Greek yogurt (or dairy-free yogurt)
- 1/2 cup coconut water
- 1 tablespoon honey or maple syrup (optional, for added sweetness)
- Handful of ice cubes

Instructions:

1. Place all ingredients in a blender.
2. Blend until smooth and creamy.
3. Taste and add honey or maple syrup if desired for sweetness.
4. Pour into glasses and serve chilled.

Nutritional Information (per serving):

- Calories: 180
- Protein: 6g
- Fat: 1g
- Carbohydrates: 35g
- Fiber: 5g
- Sugars: 25g

2. Pineapple Papaya Protein Power Smoothie

Ingredients:

- 1 cup chopped pineapple
- 1 cup chopped papaya
- 1/2 cup Greek yogurt (or dairy-free yogurt)
- 1 scoop vanilla protein powder
- 1/2 cup coconut water
- Handful of ice cubes

Instructions:

1. Add all ingredients to a blender.
2. Blend until smooth and creamy.
3. Pour into glasses and enjoy immediately.

Nutritional Information (per serving):

- Calories: 220
- Protein: 20g
- Fat: 1g
- Carbohydrates: 35g
- Fiber: 6g

- Sugars: 25g

3. Pineapple Papaya Green Goddess Smoothie

Ingredients:

- 1 cup chopped pineapple
- 1 cup chopped papaya
- 1 cup spinach leaves
- 1/2 cup Greek yogurt (or dairy-free yogurt)
- 1/2 cup coconut water
- Handful of ice cubes

Instructions:

1. Combine all ingredients in a blender.
2. Blend until smooth and creamy.
3. Pour into glasses and serve chilled.

Nutritional Information (per serving):

- Calories: 200
- Protein: 7g
- Fat: 1g
- Carbohydrates: 35g
- Fiber: 7g
- Sugars: 25g

4. Pineapple Papaya Coconut Bliss Smoothie

Ingredients:

- 1 cup chopped pineapple
- 1 cup chopped papaya
- 1/2 cup Greek yogurt (or dairy-free yogurt)
- 1/2 cup coconut milk
- Handful of ice cubes

Instructions:

1. Place all ingredients in a blender.
2. Blend until smooth and creamy.
3. Pour into glasses and garnish with shredded coconut.

Nutritional Information (per serving):

- Calories: 190
- Protein: 6g
- Fat: 5g
- Carbohydrates: 35g
- Fiber: 6g
- Sugars: 25g

5. Pineapple Papaya Citrus Zing Smoothie

Ingredients:

- 1 cup chopped pineapple
- 1 cup chopped papaya
- Juice of 1/2 orange
- 1/2 cup Greek yogurt (or dairy-free yogurt)
- 1/2 cup coconut water
- Handful of ice cubes

Instructions:

1. Add all ingredients to a blender.
2. Blend until smooth and creamy.
3. Pour into glasses and garnish with a slice of orange.

Nutritional Information (per serving):

- Calories: 180
- Protein: 6g
- Fat: 1g
- Carbohydrates: 35g
- Fiber: 6g
- Sugars: 25g

These Pineapple Papaya Paradise smoothie variations offer a tropical fusion with enzyme-rich fruits, perfect for promoting digestive ease, especially for those managing hiatal hernia symptoms. Bursting with the flavors of pineapple and papaya, these smoothies provide a delicious and soothing option to support digestive health and overall well-being. Incorporate these refreshing blends into your daily routine for a nourishing and satisfying treat.

CHAPTER FIVE
ADDITIONAL TIPS FOR DIGESTIVE WELLNESS

Incorporating Mindful Eating Practices: Listening to Your Body and Managing Stress

Mindful eating is a practice that involves paying attention to the present moment and being fully engaged in the act of eating. For individuals managing hiatal hernia and digestive discomfort, incorporating mindful eating practices can be incredibly beneficial in promoting digestive wellness and overall well-being. By tuning into your body's signals and managing stress levels, you can cultivate a more harmonious relationship with food and support your digestive health.

Listening to Your Body

One of the key principles of mindful eating is listening to your body's hunger and fullness cues. Instead of eating on autopilot or according to external cues, such as the time of day or the size of a portion, take the time to tune into your body's signals before, during, and after meals. Pay attention to sensations of hunger and satiety and honor your body's natural signals by eating when you're hungry and stopping when you're satisfied. By eating in alignment with your body's needs, you can prevent overeating and reduce the risk of digestive discomfort associated with hiatal hernia.

Additionally, practicing mindful eating can help you become more attuned to how different foods affect your body. Notice how certain foods make you feel energized and satisfied, while others may leave you feeling sluggish or uncomfortable. By becoming more aware of these subtle cues, you can make informed choices about the foods that best support your digestive health and overall well-being.

Managing Stress

Stress can have a significant impact on digestive health, exacerbating symptoms of hiatal hernia such as heartburn, acid reflux, and indigestion. Incorporating stress management techniques into your daily routine can help alleviate tension in the body and promote relaxation, which can in turn support digestive wellness.

There are many effective strategies for managing stress, and it's important to find what works best for you. Some individuals may find relief through practices such as mindfulness meditation, deep breathing exercises, or progressive muscle relaxation. Others may benefit from engaging in activities that bring them joy and relaxation, such as spending time in nature, practicing yoga, or engaging in creative pursuits.

It's also important to identify and address sources of stress in your life, whether they're related to work, relationships, or other aspects of daily life. By taking proactive steps to manage stress and cultivate a sense of calm and balance, you can support your digestive health and overall well-being.

In addition to dietary modifications, lifestyle factors play a crucial role in managing hiatal hernia and supporting digestive wellness. By incorporating healthy habits into your daily routine, you can help alleviate symptoms of hiatal hernia and promote optimal digestive function.

Exercise

Regular physical activity is essential for maintaining overall health and well-being, including digestive health. Exercise helps stimulate digestion, improve circulation, and reduce stress levels, all of which can benefit individuals managing hiatal hernia symptoms. Aim for at least 30 minutes of moderate intensity exercise most days of the week, such as brisk walking, swimming, cycling, or yoga. Choose activities that you enjoy and that feel good for your body and listen to your body's signals to avoid overexertion.

It's important to note that certain types of exercise may exacerbate symptoms of hiatal hernia, particularly activities that involve intense abdominal contractions or bending forward, such as crunches or heavy lifting. If you experience discomfort during exercise, modify your routine to focus on low-impact activities that are gentle on the digestive system.

Posture

Poor posture can contribute to hiatal hernia symptoms by putting pressure on the abdomen and exacerbating acid reflux and heartburn. Maintaining good posture throughout the day can help alleviate these symptoms and support optimal digestive function. Practice sitting and standing up straight, with your shoulders back and your spine aligned. Avoid slouching or slumping forward, especially while eating or engaging in activities that may exacerbate symptoms. Using supportive cushions or pillows to prop yourself up can also help reduce pressure on the abdomen and promote better posture.

Sleep Hygiene

Quality sleep is essential for overall health and well-being, including digestive health. Poor sleep can disrupt digestion and exacerbate symptoms of hiatal hernia, such as acid reflux and heartburn. Prioritize good sleep hygiene practices to ensure restful and rejuvenating sleep each night. Establish a regular sleep schedule by going to bed and waking up at the same time each day, even on weekends. Create a relaxing bedtime routine to signal to your body that it's time to wind down, such as taking a warm bath, reading a book, or practicing relaxation techniques. Create a sleep-friendly environment by keeping your bedroom cool, dark, and quiet, and avoiding screens and stimulating activities before bedtime.

By incorporating these lifestyle modifications into your daily routine, you can support digestive wellness and alleviate symptoms of hiatal hernia. By practicing mindful eating, managing stress, engaging in regular exercise, maintaining good posture, and prioritizing quality sleep, you can optimize your digestive health and overall well-being.

CONCLUSION

In conclusion, navigating life with hiatal hernia can present its challenges, but armed with the right knowledge and tools, you can take charge of your journey towards digestive wellness. Throughout this cookbook, we've explored the intricacies of hiatal hernia and how dietary modifications, particularly through the incorporation of smoothies, can significantly alleviate symptoms and enhance overall well-being.

From understanding the condition to discovering the benefits of smoothies and learning about essential ingredients, we've covered a wide array of topics aimed at empowering you to make informed choices for your health. Whether it's sipping on a refreshing Pineapple Papaya Paradise or indulging in a soothing Mango Coconut Cream, each smoothie variation offers a delicious and nourishing way to support digestive comfort.

Furthermore, we've delved into additional tips for digestive wellness, emphasizing the importance of mindful eating practices, stress management, exercise, posture, and sleep hygiene. By incorporating these lifestyle modifications into your daily routine, you can further enhance the efficacy of dietary interventions and optimize your digestive health.

Ultimately, this cookbook serves as a comprehensive guide and a source of empowerment on your hiatal hernia journey. By embracing the healing power of food and adopting a holistic approach to wellness, you can reclaim control over your digestive health and live a life free from discomfort and limitations.

Remember, every sip of a nutrient-packed smoothie is a step towards a healthier, happier you. Empower yourself through diet and let your journey to digestive wellness begin.

Hiatal Hernia Diet Cheat Sheet: Handy List of Foods to Enjoy and Avoid

Managing hiatal hernia symptoms through diet can be made simpler with a handy cheat sheet outlining foods to enjoy and those to avoid. This quick reference guide empowers individuals to make informed dietary choices that support digestive health and alleviate discomfort associated with hiatal hernia.

Foods to Enjoy

1. **Lean Proteins**: Opt for lean protein sources such as skinless poultry, fish, tofu, and legumes. These options provide essential nutrients without adding unnecessary fat or acidity to meals, making them gentle on the digestive system.

2. **Non-Acidic Fruits**: Choose non-acidic fruits like bananas, melons, apples, and pears. These fruits are less likely to trigger acid reflux or heartburn, making them suitable choices for individuals managing hiatal hernia symptoms.

3. **Non-Citrus Juices**: Select non-citrus juices such as apple juice, pear juice, or coconut water. These beverages offer hydration and flavor without the acidity found in citrus juices, which can aggravate symptoms of hiatal hernia.

4. **Whole Grains**: Incorporate whole grains like brown rice, quinoa, oats, and whole wheat bread into your diet. These fiber-rich foods promote digestive health and provide sustained energy, helping to prevent digestive discomfort.

5. **Low-Fat Dairy**: Choose low-fat dairy options such as skim milk, yogurt, and cheese. These dairy products offer calcium and protein without the added fat that can exacerbate symptoms of hiatal hernia.

6. **Vegetables**: Enjoy a variety of vegetables, focusing on non-acidic options like leafy greens, carrots, cucumbers, and sweet potatoes. These vegetables are rich in vitamins, minerals, and fiber, supporting overall digestive wellness.

Foods to Avoid

1. **High-Fat Foods**: Limit high-fat foods such as fried foods, fatty cuts of meat, and rich desserts. These foods can relax the lower esophageal sphincter (LES) and increase the risk of acid reflux and heartburn.

2. **Acidic Fruits**: Avoid acidic fruits like citrus fruits, tomatoes, and pineapples. These fruits can trigger acid reflux and exacerbate symptoms of hiatal hernia, leading to discomfort and irritation.

3. **Citrus Juices**: Steer clear of citrus juices such as orange juice, grapefruit juice, and lemonade. These beverages are highly acidic and can worsen symptoms of acid reflux and heartburn.

4. **Carbonated Beverages**: Limit carbonated beverages like soda and sparkling water. The bubbles in these drinks can expand in the stomach, putting pressure on the LES and increasing the likelihood of acid reflux.

5. **Spicy Foods**: Avoid spicy foods such as chili peppers, hot sauces, and spicy curries. These foods can irritate the esophagus and exacerbate

symptoms of hiatal hernia, leading to discomfort and inflammation.

6. **Alcohol and Caffeine**: Reduce or eliminate alcohol and caffeine from your diet, as they can relax the LES and promote acid reflux. Instead, opt for non-alcoholic and caffeine-free alternatives to support digestive health.

By referencing this handy cheat sheet, individuals managing hiatal hernia can make mindful food choices that support digestive wellness and alleviate discomfort. With a focus on incorporating nutrient-rich foods while avoiding triggers, individuals can take control of their diet and enhance their quality of life.

Creating hiatal hernia-friendly smoothies is made easier with a substitution guide that offers alternatives for common ingredients based on dietary needs. Whether your lactose intolerant, following a vegan diet, or have specific preferences, these substitutions ensure that everyone can enjoy delicious and nourishing smoothies tailored to their individual needs.

Dairy Substitutions

1. **Non-Dairy Milk**: Replace dairy milk with non-dairy alternatives such as almond milk, coconut milk, soy milk, or oat milk. These options provide a creamy texture and rich flavor without the lactose found in dairy milk, making them suitable for individuals with lactose intolerance or dairy allergies.

2. **Dairy-Free Yogurt**: Opt for dairy-free yogurt made from coconut milk, almond milk, or soy milk. These alternatives offer the probiotic benefits of traditional yogurt without the dairy content, making them suitable for individuals following a vegan or dairy-free diet.

3. **Plant-Based Protein Powder**: Choose plant-based protein powders made from sources such as pea protein, hemp protein, or brown rice protein. These options offer a complete protein source without the whey or casein found in traditional protein powders, catering to individuals with dairy allergies or dietary restrictions.

Sweeteners Substitutions

1. **Maple Syrup**: Substitute maple syrup with honey, agave nectar, or date syrup. These natural sweeteners offer a rich flavor and smooth texture without the fructose content found in maple syrup, making them suitable for individuals looking to reduce their sugar intake.

2. **Stevia**: Opt for stevia or monk fruit extract as a calorie-free alternative to traditional sweeteners. These options provide sweetness without the glycemic impact of sugar, making them suitable for individuals following a low-carbohydrate or diabetic-friendly diet.

3. **Fruit**: Use ripe bananas, dates, or berries to naturally sweeten smoothies. These fruits offer natural sugars and fiber, providing sweetness and texture without the need for added sweeteners.

Ingredient Substitutions

1. **Leafy Greens**: Substitute spinach with kale, Swiss chard, or collard greens. These leafy greens offer similar nutritional benefits and can be used interchangeably in smoothie recipes.

2. **Frozen Fruit**: Use fresh fruit as an alternative to frozen fruit in smoothies. Simply wash and chop fresh fruit before adding it to the blender, adjusting the amount of ice or liquid as needed to achieve the desired consistency.

3. **Nut Butter**: Replace peanut butter with almond butter, cashew butter, or sunflower seed butter. These options offer a creamy texture and rich flavor without the potential allergens found in peanuts,

making them suitable for individuals with nut allergies.

By referencing this smoothie ingredient substitution guide, individuals can customize their smoothie recipes to accommodate their dietary needs and preferences. Whether your lactose intolerant, vegan, or simply looking to reduce your sugar intake, these alternatives ensure that everyone can enjoy delicious and nourishing smoothies tailored to their individual needs.